SPACES BETWEEN US

SPACES BETWEEN US

POETRY, PROSE AND ART ON HIV/AIDS

Edited by

Kelly Norman Ellis | M. L. Hunter

TWP
THIRD WORLD PRESS
Progressive Black Publishing Since 1967
Chicago, IL

Third World Press
Publishers since 1967
Chicago

First Edition
Printed in the United States of America

Front cover painting Love Potion © by Christopher Jarred; photographed by Glodean Champion
Back cover painting A.I.D.S. (Africa is Dying Swiftly) © by Ghariokwu Lemi
Cover design and interior layout by Denise Borel Billups
Text set in Filosofia Regular

ISBN13: 978-0-88378-320-7
Library of Congress Control Number: 2009941522

Artwork:
Page 1: Untitled © by Viet Lê
Page 20: A.I.D.S. (Africa is Dying Swiftly) © by Ghariokwu Lemi
Page 31: A Long Ride To Nowhere © by Geoffrey D. Holman
Page 51: Please Take a Ticket © by Richard Sawdon Smith
Page 61: Untitled © by Viet Lê
Page 65: Recover/Discover © by Richard Sawdon Smith
Page 67: Protest © by Cyrille Phipps
Page 84: Positive Voices of Dorm E © by Rural Women's Health Project
Page 101: Title Card © by Cyrille Phipps
Page 110: Doctor, One Day I Found a Cure © by Michelle Mashon
Page 140: Web of Life © by Roopali Kambo
Page 141: Untitled © by Viet Lê
Page 179: Absent Body © by Richard Sawdon Smith
Page 202: Social Conscious III © by Ronnie Queenan

All about are the cold places,
all about are the pushmen and jeopardy, theft—
all about are the stormers and scramblers but
what must our Season be, which starts from Fear?
Live and go out.
Define and
medicate the whirlwind.

Gwendolyn Brooks
from "The Second Sermon on the Warpland"

Contents

SECTION II
VIGIL

SECTION III
LIVE ONE MORE DAY

I AM

H.Y.P.E. Spring 2009 Troupe

I...

I...

I...

I am ...

I am ...

I am ...

I am HIV.

I am HIV.

I am HIV.

And ...

Introduction

Kelly Norman Ellis

When I moved to Chicago eleven years ago, I rode the El everywhere. I loved watching the people. I remember a ride from Hyde Park to Oak Lawn on a fall day. I watched as college students and professors entered the cars. As we moved through Chinatown, folks crowded on with packages, then to the Loop with its neatly coiffed businessmen and women. On and on it went. The working class, the poor, the wealthy, children, and the elderly moved in and out. I heard Mississippi accents, Spanish, and languages I did not recognize. And we sat next to each other. Our bodies so close. Almost touching. Most of the time we did not make eye contact. Even if the train was crowded with bodies, and we accidently touched, we pretended not to feel. We pretended we were alone.

I thought of these train rides when I read Emanuel Xavier's beautiful poem "Cielo." His lines, "Like the sky above, I want to span the spaces between us/from Bushwick to Aztlan," moved me as I read the submissions for this anthology. I kept coming back to this poem, this articulation of space. I knew these words were the heart of the project. In 2009, it is no secret that HIV and AIDS is global. This disease cares nothing about sexuality, gender, race, ethnicity, or religion as it invades the blood. One of the reasons I believe this disease thrives is our inability to fully understand our common humanity. In our pain, we want to blame others for this disease. *Gay men and the down low, drug addicts, risky lifestyles.* I remember in the early 1990s the expression innocent victims of AIDS. Who is the innocent victim? Who is the guilty victim? I have grown tired of us fighting each other. In the pages of this book are women and men living with this disease, gay and straight, Latino, Black, and Asian. They are from the United States, Jamaica, India, and Mexico. They want us to survive, all of us.

For all the people I know living with this disease with support and love, I hear stories of those who die alone without family or loved ones to hold on to because we fill the spaces between us with shame and fear. What would happen if we realized that we are all living with HIV/ AIDS? We have all lost our fathers, sisters, brothers, cousins, mothers, babies, uncles, aunts, and friends to this disease. HIV and AIDS should not break the sacred bonds that hold us. We should hold on tighter to each other. We can and should touch each other. We are all trying to live, those with the virus in their blood and those who love those people.

M.L. Hunter and I wanted to create a healing space in this collection: a space to remember the sacredness of all our lives ("God is in the Particles They Say"), to remember the dead ("Vigil") and to celebrate the work it takes to survive ("Live One More Day"). Fear is no longer an option. We have too much work to do, too many people who need to stay alive. We must always acknowledge the hell of this disease, remember the ones we have lost to it and fight to fill the spaces between us with the healing balms of compassion and love.

M. L. Hunter

How has HIV become normal? Better yet, is HIV normal? Before the World Wide Web and twenty-four hour news coverage there was a disease that did not have a name, but according to our news outlets at the time, it had a targeted population — white gay men. Not just any white gay men; this untitled killer was primarily on the west and east coast in America according to CBS, ABC, CBS, *Time, Newsweek* ...you get the picture. The Midwest was safe. One thing that is true about being human, or at least those who are part of popular American culture, is sensationalism ties us together. What can we talk about around the water cooler at work the next day is what drives us.

When gay white were mysteriously dying from what was labeled as GRID (gay-related immune deficiency), the general public had nothing to concern itself with. We were safe as long as we were not involved in homosexual activities. As a student at Thomas Carr Howe High School (Indianapolis), we had to read *Time* magazine as part of a civics class; we also had to watch the evening news. This was to help teach us how the world is held together. By the time I finished my senior year, I felt comfortable with Americanized news and it played a significant role when members of the Class of 1986 were passing around our senior memory books. Besides the pictures, notes, and all the pop culture there was one section that has stayed with me — news stories. What were the biggest local, national, and international stories? I will have to go pull out my senior book to quote the international story (I believe it centered on terrorism), but the national and local story could easily serve as international stories. The explosion of the Space Shuttle was the first "where were you" scenario in my life. That day I happened to be on a field trip visiting the City-County building in downtown Indianapolis learning how the judicial system operated. Members of my class were standing behind a judge watching the procedures when the announcement was made. The local story reaches outside of Indianapolis to Kokomo, Indiana — Ryan White. The boy who received what was once GRID and now HIV from a blood transfusion. So, with Ryan's story did we miss the marker this immune attacking disease could reach any of us?

We continued to watch and read news stories about the virus that seemed to have no end. But medication would come to help and through my undergrad years in the Indiana University system, I would see example after example of people with tables filled with drugs to help keep them alive. Without being aware, we were being sensitized to HIV. The only downfall was men who have sex with men (gay, down low, same-gender loving, homosexual, queer...) were left holding the bag. It worked. Another stereotype was born.

Larry, the first person I was mutually in love with told me, "everyone is going to get this disease (HIV)." I was 24 trying to make my way in life, in New York City, and did not want to believe him. Not everyone was going to get this disease. Looking back, my subconscious was programmed by my pop culture news media – only homosexuals will get the virus and anyone else who gets it outside of this arena were just a by-product that could be directly linked back to a gay root. That was 1993. Like my senior book, Larry's words stay with me, but I could not let that hinder me from exploring freedom to make my own choices, including sex. As I entered my adult life and the sexually transmitted disease of the day was HIV and there was no cure.

Just like the freedom I began to explore in my life, HIV was doing the same; only in a bigger way. This virus went on a worldwide tour and has been hosted at all levels of society. Magic Johnson told the world of his infection; Arthur Ashe died from AIDS related complication; Easy-E vanished right before the Hip-Hop/Rap world. Young girls who are virgins in parts of Africa have been demoralized because of the belief an HIV infected person having sex with a virgin would cure them. There was a time in India when the virus was able to be tracked by the trucking route through the country. Was Larry right and the pretty stereotype for understanding by media about HIV wrong?

The major changing year for HIV was 1996 when Dr. David Ho was *Time* magazine's Person of the Year for developing the "cocktail" therapy for HIV. That year was the initial turning point; HIV was no longer news worthy. White gay men had advocated to the point where they influenced governmental policies on all levels and they wrote their own paychecks to start agencies and careers in HIV.

The number of women becoming infected continued to increase and infection rates exploded for Black gay men without fanfare. My friend Umar Hasan in his poem "The Day Hurricane Elisa Hit Home" said it best: "The world didn't stand still that day, it just/ walked on by."

There is one important aspect when discussing HIV; the "H" has been neglected time and time again. The immunodeficiency virus part may not be a layman's term, but the effects are. Standing around water coolers has been replaced by bottled water, but for a disease that has no cure, but does have treatments helping to make it chronic, we are more concerned about how someone became infected than the fact it is not targeted to any population other than human. *Spaces Between Us* voices the pain, anger, fear, and hope that continue to exist.

Section I

God's in the Particles They Say

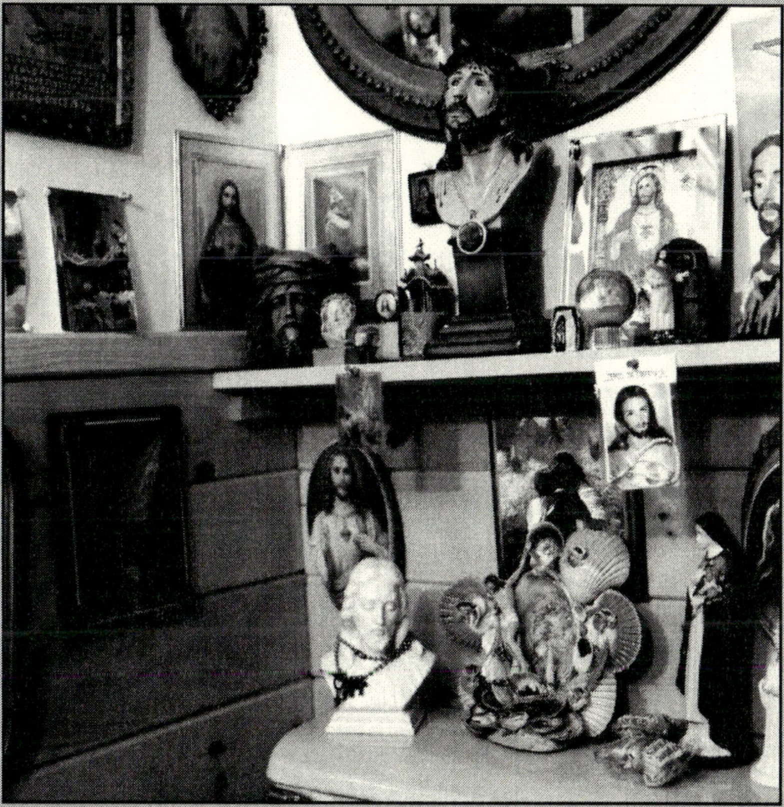

Untitled | **Viet Lê**

Elegy for a Trojan

Samantha Thornhill

Latex moon
rising in the sky
of my sex,
the night we met my
hyena streaked the sheets
with untamed
glee-ooh we!

Since the day
I watched you
swallow whole my health
teacher's eggplant
I have breathed
your name.

Citizen of Troy
fallen in flame,
I've scanned
your tragic tale.
Of your plight I'll say it
plain: you got fucked.

So tell me, how
many times
have you spared me
from hollow stallions
brimming with deadly

little men?
Too flushed
you are
to say. Hell.
I wouldn't
believe you
anyway, Pinocchio—
pancake flip
pinch your tip and
watch your nose grow.

Caught on floors
of the responsibly
misbehaved,
billboarding left eyes back when
TLC first raged—this

I know: you
left my body
intact with tailed
tragedies in tow,

lengthened
yourself to lengthen
my days.

But don't nobody
love you when
you broke.
The morning after
you did, down slid

an atomic pill
detonating deep
within my ecology.

Old friend,
consider this
an apology wrapped
in so long ,
resting on a silver tray.

Trojan, I regret
to confess,
there were times
I felt
only you
in the dark.

And we have
been strangers too,
more,
more,
than I can say

the layin up: monroe on layin down with ari

avery r young

we blendin browns; twistin ourselves dizzy inside luther lyrics n sandlewood incense. we chicken grease; dat damn nigga johnson or oooo weee robinson naked n guilt free. we make believin we aint lethal in order to engage in full fledge high noon freakyness, searchin tongues fo sense of anything — love or first names not included. we cool wid bein red of darkrooms, n right here right when right now mean erything, we be two with an issue of blood surfin de multitude yearnin to touch de hem of our garments. we be back in de days on de boulevard of ashe, wright n kuti. we spittin fact; praticin faith, somethin like nmemenon. we saturday skin on top of sunday sin, underneath raincoat hooks n timberland boot boxes. *we commere n lemme find out what dat good-good hit fo.* we music; chest crashin back; kneecaps gainst thigh; lips smackin neck;and cheek scrapin naps. even wid our eyes open we sound like earth, wind n throbbin dicks, hopin our dirty talk match our do me baby. we wanna stop to figure out what part of africa be in our nose width n jawlines, but archeology n physical education two different sciences. n we gotta be bout de bidness of configurin us, tumblin into somethin thick n meaningless. inside dis moment, we what we ever wanted to do n did, but never ourselves n dats why we sad. leanin tward lost, leakin loneliness through pores so open n shameful we know better than to look back. we savin ourselves from becomin salt or sorry, or de elephant tween our embrace. we dont wanna wish we cud get up, dress ourselves, play patty cake n go to no place like home. we wanna stay de way we entered dis life, play find my spot n lay yo weight on it five minutes longer dan de luther lyrics n sandlewood incense can keep a room from tellin our ears n noses what we are doin. n we wanna shoot de sky a pretty sticky circumstance. right here, right when right now means we are bein held accountable fo way mo than we could ever carry on our strongest backs. we refuse to fold, or cry, or sneeze. we link up, become back in de days on de boulevard of hughes, baldwin n cullen; n we get able to hold we high n steady. de pressure to stay locked in dis pleasure will kill us way befo de raw fuk will.

The Day Of the Dead

E. J. Guarino

Jack's mother stared out the window of her son's hospital room at a city shrouded in white. At 11:10 AM there had been a few random flakes. By 11:20, snow was falling steadily; and within another fifteen minutes it was coming down with a vengeance, covering everything. Nothing has been spared, she thought. It was a view that underscored the bleakness of her situation: her son was dying; of that there was no question. From the eleventh floor of Cabrini Medical Center she had a far-reaching view, but she could not see what her son was seeing.

> *The angel stood poised above the marble slab, wings spread, one finger pressed against its lips in a gesture of silence. Then, lowering its hand it pointed downward and Jack saw engraved in stone:*
>
> *Joaquin Jacobo*
> *January 4, 1953 -*

Jack sat upright in bed, startling his mother. He was drenched in sweat and gasping for air.

"*¿Mijo, que te pasa?*"

"*Nada, nada*, just a bad dream." He brought his breathing back to normal as quickly as he could and even managed a smile. He did not want to worry his mother more. She was already upset as it was. Had he fooled her? He wasn't sure. He had never managed it as a child, but he had learned that his mother sometimes let him believe he had. Which was it now, he wondered. It was always hard to tell what was on her mind if that was the way she wanted it. At other times it was all too clear what she was thinking. But now, she wasn't quite herself. She sat in the chair closest to his bed and read or looked out the window. When she spoke it was consciously about inconsequential things so Jack would have no idea just how difficult this trip had been for her.

She had flown from Mexico City to be with her son, but she felt alone. To her, the only difference between New York and Sodom and Gommorah was that one had a subway. The city intimidated her. The buildings, so tall and crowded together, seemed like angry fists raised in defiance. No charm, she thought. Where is this city's charm? Where is its humanity? It has none, she concluded. Not like *La Capital. Ay, La Capital!*

As she drifted into a reverie about the delights of her beloved *Ciudad de Mexico*, she would remember the reason she had come to this cold *ciudad norteamericana.* It was because of the terrible disease, the one whose name she could not even bring herself to say. If my son has to die why couldn't it be from some respectable sickness like cancer? Such ideas were uneducated, she knew, but she could not help thinking them. Feeling guilty, she would stroke her son's hand saying, "*Mi pobre niño,*" and busy herself with fussing over him, anything to stop such unmotherly thoughts.

Señora Jacobo had never approved of her son's decision to leave Mexico; the direction his art had taken; his life, in general; and the nature of his dying, in particular. What would people say! But she was his mother and, no matter what, she was determined to stand by him. Isn't that, after all, what a mother is for? And to herself she said over and over, "*Soy una mujer con studios.*" As if doing so would drive the demons away.

She had taken a leave from her teaching position and had flown to *Los Estados Unidos* alone since her husband refused to join her. She had tried to convince him to make the trip with her, but after much arguing, he had exploded with his final say on the matter: "As he lived, let him die."

"*Debes de tener verguenza,*" had been Senora Jacobo's cold reply. As she packed, her husband ranted, "*Si*, shame! Now, you understand!" But she did not; neither did he. There had been nothing more to say on the subject. She had left hoping that he might reconsider but knew in her deepest heart he would not.

Señora Jacobo had been to New York before, in happier times but, even then, she had not really warmed to the city. She spoke English well, and with each visit there always seemed to be more Spanish speaking people. But something was missing; exactly what she wasn't sure, but she knew it wasn't there just the same. Perhaps it was a heart. *Si*, this was *una ciudad sin corazon.* How could this be? Her Joaquin, her heart, was here. Such foolishness! *No es importante.* Then she would force herself to think of other things.

She had been here a month in this cold northern city. She spent each day in the hospital and before dark walked to Jack's Greenwich Village studio apartment. She shunned the subway as too confusing and oppressive. She was not able to travel on it with the ease she was used to on *El Metro* back home. So, after a few attempts, she gave up in frustration and disgust, preferring the sureness of her own two feet. Sometimes she would pray at the Church of Our Lady of Pompeii on Carmine Street, only a block away from the apartment, but she did not really feel at home in this Italian church, as she thought of it. She longed for churches with familiar names like Santo Domingo, San Francisco, and San Juan de Dios. Instead, whenever possible, she went to Nuestra Señora de Guadalupe on West 14th Street to ask the Virgin for help.

"*Ayudame, Madre.* Save my son. And help me in this heartless place. I don't know what to do. I want to go home; this is too painful. Why is this happening to me? I'm frightened. A son should not die before his mother; you of all people should know that. *Ay, Dios mio. Disculpame.* Forgive me for thinking only of myself."

Each day in the hospital she saw her son weakening, and each week he lost more weight. Always there seemed to be a new complication. It broke her heart to look at him, but she could not let him see this. He was her youngest, her baby. How could this be happening? Why him? She stared out the window again.

"*¿Mama?*"

"*¿Que te pasa, Joaquin?*"

"Jack, mama. Jack.

"*Joaquin,*" his mother said firmly, but with a slight smile, indicating there would be nothing more said on this topic.

She tolerated many things, but not this. She had never forgiven her son for changing his name, but after many years and many more arguments "this thing of the name," as they came to refer to it, had become an affectionate sort of game between them, though neither's opinion had changed.

"Are you alright, *mijo*?"

"Just a little tired. Same as usual. It's getting late. You look exhausted. Why don't you go home."

"In a little while."

If only I could go home, she thought. But she couldn't say this to her son. Home to him was his little apartment; for her it was much more. For Jack, home had become an apartment decorated in what he considered the American style. It had been important that it reflect his adopted country: the walls were hung with prints of paintings from the Hudson School, photos of New York in the early 1900s, and reproductions of photographs by Ansel Adams and Edwin S. Curtis cut from magazines. Furniture consisted of two Shaker-style chairs, a trunk, an old wooden table salvaged from a second hand store and a daybed over which lay Jack's prize possession—a quilt with the tree of life design. Reminders of his homeland were few but meaningful: a picture of the Virgin of Guadalupe in a tin frame; a black pot from Oaxaca; and a Day of the Dead figure, its arms and legs tiny springs, which he had found as a teenager in a shop in Puerto Vallarta. For his mother, home meant family, church, and country. Jack sensed that his mother felt lost, but said nothing. Neither would talk about it for fear of upsetting the other and, instead, long silences settled in. Jack was tired and afraid to close his eyes for fear of dreaming again, but after a few minutes of resistance, he gave in.

Standing next to his bed, the angel touched him gently on the shoulder. He beckoned to him. Jack felt as if he were slipping deeper underwater. He struggled, but felt himself pulled downward. He was making no headway. He grew tired, but with one final effort, broke the surface and inhaled.

"*¿Que te pasa? ¿Que te pasa?*"

"Just another bad dream. Don't worry. I'll be alright." But jack was breathing heavily, his eyes wide with fear. His mother turned away from him and, looked out the window again. Somehow doing so gave her a sense of freedom, a place for her mind to escape from what she knew she would eventually have to face but not now, not now.

"This is too difficult, too difficult," she said not so much to her son but more out of a need to express out loud her feeling that what was happening to her son was not only unjust; it was cruel, too heavy a cross to bear.

"Do you think this is easy for me? I'm the one going through it. How do you think I feel? I know how this ends; I've been through it before. Do you know how many friends I've watched die? Fifteen! I've lost fifteen friends, *mama*, and I've lost track of how many acquaintances have died. They were men with their whole lives ahead of them, and then, suddenly, they had to face things they should never have even known about. They became shriveled and old before their time. Their conversations were a strange alphabet of illnesses and treatments: CMV, AZT, MRI. So don't tell me how difficult this is, *mama*, because you don't want to face it. I can't look away. I don't have that luxury, not anymore."

"What can I say, *mijo*? My heart is breaking." As she said these words she saw a look of panic come over her son's face. "*¿Que te pasa? ¿Que te pasa?*"

Jack whispered, "*Mama*, I've soiled myself."

It happened five more times that night, and each time the nurse was called Jack became more terrified, and his mother became increasingly worried. She would not leave the hospital this night, she knew. Finally, her son was put into diapers causing Esperanza Jacobo to think: He is truly my baby again. Oh, how this disease mocks us!

With each of these incidents Jack became weaker and more silent. Near dawn, just before he fell asleep, Jack turned to his mother and said, "In this country, *mama*, they always talk of death with dignity; it's a very popular notion, you know; but this doesn't seem very dignified to me."

"*Mijo*, we struggle to get into this world; we struggle to live in it and, I guess, we must struggle to leave it."

As her son fell asleep, Señora Jacobo watched him from her usual place, the chair next to his bed, and remembered the day she had arrived from Mexico. She had been startled by her son's frailty; he had once been so robust, so alive! Jack had been muscular like the men he photographed, but his booming voice and hearty, infectious laugh were his most memorable attributes. Now his shiny, black hair was thin and gray and he walked with much difficulty, connected to an IV pole. The first time he had broken into a severe sweat she had helped him change his pajamas, and was shocked by the tube protruding from his chest.

"What's that?" she had asked.

"A Hickman catheter. It makes it easier for them to give me medicine," Jack had calmly replied.

Her son had then told her that he was losing his sight, but that there was some hope that it could be saved. She had then reached out and gently touched the tubing. Over the weeks she had been with her son she had watched him steadily deteriorate. His eyes had been stabilized, but his vision was so poor that it would be difficult, if not impossible, for him to work as a photographer again. As Jack grew weaker he became more sullen.

"I've got to get out of here. I've got work to do," was something Jack began to say often, but Señora Jacobo was careful not to respond, preferring silence to argument. She did not approve of much of her son's photographic work, and Jack was well aware of her opinion. *No need to go into all of that again, especially now,* each thought. Many of the photographs depicted muscular men — alone, in couples, or in groups — in striking poses, nude or wearing little more than small loincloths and elaborate Mayan or Aztec headdresses. The eroticism was palpable and, although Jack photographed urban landscapes, bucolic scenes, and, now and then, a still life, it was his exotic photographs of men, which had recently caught the attention of influential collectors. None of this impressed Señora Jacobo.

After one of her son's many complaints that he should be working, Señora Jacobo at last ventured to say something.

"*Mijo, no es importante.* Your health must come first."

"My work was never important to you," her son snapped.

She tried to explain, but Jack refused to listen and ranted on.

"My work is not just what I do; it's who I am," he shouted. "You can't accept that because you can't accept me."

"It doesn't seem right to me," she said softly. You're my son and I love you; I wouldn't be here if I didn't, *pero no comprendo tu vida.* I just don't understand."

"You don't have to understand — anymore than I understand your life. My whole life I had to pretend; that's why I left Mexico. I don't pretend anymore."

There was silence then between mother and son; not the silence of anger, not even the silence of hurt. It was just that neither wanted to say more on this subject. They had, after all, said these things to each other before; why do so again.

It was painful for Señora Jacobo to recall what had happened, and even more so to contemplate what was to come. Looking down now at her sleeping child she thought: *What next, my son? What next?*

Señora Jacobo was a petite woman who looked even smaller in the oversized reclining chair that the hospital supplied, which had become her bed. She went back to Jack's apartment early each afternoon for a bath, a change of clothes, and a quick meal; then, after carefully arranging her hair, she would hurry back to her son. Señora Jacobo always wore neatly tailored suits — jacket, blouse, skirt — in black, brown, navy, or gray. She only wore serious colors, as she thought of them, only befitting her profession; nothing frivolous would be appropriate. Over her heart she pinned her most valued possession, a cameo incised with the image of the Virgin of Guadalupe, which had been in her family for four generations. Whenever Senora Jacobo was anxious she would finger this treasure although she was totally unaware of doing so.

When winter finally turned to spring, Señora Jacobo decided to decorate Jack's room for Easter, thinking that this might cheer him up. The walls were painted a stark white and, except for a sickly green curtain which could be drawn around the bed for privacy, the room was austere and devoid of color so Señora Jacobo taped cardboard bunnies to the window and had one of the orderlies hang a few from the ceiling.

"Very American, *verdad?*"

"Very!" Jack had replied sarcastically.

Nonetheless, she decided to do much the same for any other American holiday she could think of, unaware of the macabre twist Jack would eventually give this diversion. The Stars and Stripes went up for Memorial Day and, again, for the Fourth of July. She was hard pressed to come up with something for Labor Day, but eventually settled on a combination of autumn leaves and pictures she had drawn of hammers and saws.

The summer had been difficult for Jack. The warm weather made him think of the happier times he had spent as a teenager with his family in Puerto Vallarta. Hollywood had descended on the quiet little fishing village a few years before, but hordes of foreign tourists had not yet beaten a path to its sunny shores. Jack had been enthralled by the endless stretch of ocean and sky, mountains so rugged and vividly green they seemed more imagined than real, and the flowers that bloomed everywhere. He enjoyed the relaxed way of life and had spent most of his vacation walking the beaches or exploring the countryside on horseback, on some days riding to small farms in the nearby hills of the Sierra Madre. Others were spent swimming at Los Muertos Beach and then watching the fisherman haul in the day's catch. Every so often he would borrow a small boat from one of the locals and go to Mismaloya where he would spend hours investigating the secluded cove's abandoned movie set. But most of all Jack enjoyed long walks alone along the edge of the sea. He found the silence restful, broken only by rumble and sshh of the waves as they broke against the shore — sometimes loudly, sometimes softly.

His favorite time to be near the water was sunset. Each afternoon he would hurry down to the rocky coast south of town, strip off his clothes and stretch out on one of the boulders, hands behind his head, to wait for the spectacle. He delighted in seeing the bay turn a glittering silver before being transformed into fiery gold. The sky was streaked azure, pink, and mauve as if a giant paintbrush had been dragged across it before the sun finally departed to be reborn on the morrow. It was a sight which filled Jack with intense joy and, at the same time, made him feel sad, but he didn't know why. Perched in his secret spot above the Pacific, he stared in fascination at the contours of the massive rocks, the sweep of the coastline, and how, as the sun made its slow descent to the horizon, the mountains were shaded as if sketched in charcoal. For the rest of his life, Jack had never again felt so free or so alive as when he had gazed out at the vast expanse of the Pacific, and had been surrounded by beauty and his family.

Autumn approached with its unmistakable signs: gray skies, trees bare of leaves, and a chill in the air. Jack was still in disposable diapers and, as his high fevers and sweats became more frequent, a sort of panic set into his soul. He couldn't have explained it even if he had wanted to. As far as he was concerned, it was just that he could not bear the idea of another gloomy northern winter and he was determined to escape.

One day, without any prior warning, he turned to his mother and calmly announced, "Mama, I want to go back to Puerto Vallarta."

"*Mijo,*" his mother said gently, "*no es posible.* We couldn't manage it."

"Yes. Yes, we can."

"Joaquin, be realistic! You can hardly stand much less walk; you're attached to a pole. We couldn't even make it to the airport. It can't be done. You must accept that, *mijo.*"

Ignoring his mother's words, Jack threw back the covers and attempted to get out of bed. When he realized he could not, he fell back, turned his face away from his mother and quietly cried himself to sleep.

The angel, its wings spread, stood at the foot of the bed his arms outstretched, beckoning. Frozen with fear and anger, Jack lay immobile as the angel walked to the side of the bed and turned down the covers.

"*Mama!* I saw Death. He tried to get into bed with me, but I told him 'No! Go away! I'm not ready yet!'"

"Lay back, *mijo. ¡No te agites!*"

"I hear him, *mama!* His wings! Don't you hear them?"

"It's only the pigeons outside on the windowsill, *mijo.* Calm down. Don't upset yourself."

"I'm afraid, *mama.* I'm so afraid." His voice was so weak his mother could barely hear him.

"*Si, mijo. Yo se. Esta bien.*"

"Why are you sitting so far away, mama? Come closer, I want to hold your hand."

It was not so much death that Jack feared as much as what might come after. Back home the souls of the departed had been so real they had their own feast day on which they were given a divine reprieve, and were allowed to return to earth to bask in the warmth of their families. What if everything he had ever been told was wrong? Not about the saints and God, but what if after you died there was nothing or worse what if you were all alone in darkness. Jack had never given these matters much thought but, even though they now consumed him, he could not bring himself to reveal his confusion to his mother. It was an enigma he had to solve alone.

Nurses, orderlies, aides, and doctors entered and left Jack's room with regularity, but Señora Jacobo was only barely aware of them because she was so consumed with the pain of her son's dying. Mostly she would just stare out of the window seeing little, noticing neither the skyscrapers nor the people scurrying far below them, lost in their own lives. But November brought with it the kind of surprise Esperaza Jacobo had never expected. As she entered her son's room she froze, dangling from the ceiling were dozens of cardboard skeletons. Her astonishment was compounded by the fact that her son did not look much different from the macabre figures suspended above him.

"*¡Mi muerte, mama!*" said Jack giving the traditional greeting, and expecting a "dead" in return, but his mother had been stunned into silence. When she could finally speak it was to scold him.

"*Mijo*, this is not funny."

"*Pero, mama*, this is *El Dia de Los Muertos*, the Day of the Dead. Have you forgotten? It is the day we welcome Death and laugh at him."

""How did you manage this?" A sweep of Señora Jacobo's arm indicated the skeletons.

"I got one of the orderlies to do it. I told him it was for Halloween."

"Under the circumstances, *mijo*, you'll forgive me if I don't join in your *fiesta*."

"You don't understand, *mama*. I'm not afraid anymore. Whatever is going to be is going to be, and there's no use worrying about it. I spit at Death. Once he takes me what else can he do to me? It will be a hollow victory. What will he get? A sack of bones and very little flesh as you well know."

Señora Jacobo had never heard her son talk this way. She wasn't sure if he had accepted the fact of his dying or if he was being bitter and cynical. In either case, she didn't know what to make of such talk or how to respond to it.

"There's one thing I am worried about, mama."

"What, *mijo*?"

"My photographs. If something should happen to them then I would truly be dead. I want you to promise me that you won't destroy any of them."

"*Mijo*, what do you mean?"

"You know exactly what I mean, *mama*. Promise me!"

"You know how I feel about *those* pictures, *mijo*."

"Those *photographs* are art, *mama*. You're educated. You know better — or at least you should. Promise me!"

"*No te agites. No te agites.*" Esperanza Jacobo spoke softly, trying to separate thoughts from feelings. True, certain photographs offended her, no disturbed her, but this was her dying son's wish. How could she refuse him, especially when for his entire life she could never deny him anything?

"I'll do whatever you wish, *mijo*, whatever you wish."

It seemed that November was destined to hold a number of shocks for Esperanza Jacobo. One day late in the month, she entered her son's room and her eyes went instinctively to his face. Tubes were in his nose and for a few seconds she was at a loss as to what this meant. When she had left him an hour ago to have lunch in the cafeteria he had been sleeping. Her son was on oxygen, but why? Before she could speak, however, Jack answered her question.

"I have a touch of pneumonia, *mama*. I've had it before."

"But I .... "

"You never knew because I never told you. What would have been the point when you were so far away?"

Jack didn't tell his mother that the doctors were not sure if he had pneumonia or tuberculosis; the tests hadn't come back yet. As a precaution, he was placed in isolation and a sign stating so was placed on the door to his room which now had to be kept closed at all times. Everyone who entered had to wear a medical mask and any hospital staff that came into contact with him had to wear latex gloves as well.

Jack suddenly turned to his mother and said, "I'm too young to die. I'm frightened! I'm frightened! What if I don't get better?" Except for agreeing with him she didn't know what else to say.

Esperanza Jacobo hugged her son as if she would never let go, and said very clearly into his ear, "No matter what happens, I'll be with you, *mijo.* I'll never leave you. I promise."

"I'm so tired of being sick, *mama.*"

It was unbearable to see her son with so many tubes in his body, his skin a sickly grayish hue, and his breathing labored, but Esperanza Jacobo knew it was a thing she must bear. Her son spent most of his time sleeping now, and when he woke stared out from sunken eyes as if at something no one else could see. To his mother, it seemed he had given up. A doctor (which one she could not recall) had come one day and taken her aside saying, "We've done all we can do for him." Had Jack heard? She would never know. It was hard to admit that there was no hope. Her son no longer looked like himself. His skin was drawn tightly over his bones, and when she looked at him she saw more skull than face. He was not eating or drinking and she knew he would not last much longer. She had signed the Do Not Resuscitate Order; it had been the hardest act of her life. *How can they ask a mother to do this?* She had thought. I brought him into this world. Must I now help him to leave it? How can I let him go? I can't. In the end, she had signed, as she knew she must. Jack rarely spoke now, but one night he awoke, turned to his mother and said quietly, "I'm so tired. I wish all this was over. It's hard work, you know." He had then simply fallen back to sleep and, with each passing hour, his breathing had became increasingly shallow.

There was a terrible ache in Esperanza Jacobo's heart that night. That's how she would have described it. As she held her son's hand she believed that she could feel the very warmth of life itself draining out his fingers. She wanted to whisper,

"Let go, let it end," and at the same time she wanted to cry, "Don't go! Don't leave me, *mijo!* Live!" But she could say nothing, and instead held her dying son's hand, and spoke soothingly to him of happier days in Puerto Vallarta, never knowing if he had heard her. Never in her life would Esperanza Jacobo feel as alone as she did in the middle of that night sitting in her son's darkened hospital room so far from home.

Sometime around 4:00 AM on December 12, 1993, Esperanza Jacobo woke up. The room was dark except for a small light over the bed that illuminated her son's face. She was still holding his hand with her forehead pressed against it. Jack's eyes fluttered open briefly and, before slipping under the peaceful waves of what seemed to be a heavy sleep, he saw standing behind his mother the angel. As Esperanza Jacobo looked up it seemed to her that a smile flickered across her son's face. She could not be sure, but for the rest of her life she would take comfort from the thought that at that precise moment in time it had.

The town glowed with sunlight as Jack ran through the cobblestone streets, peering into windows and doorways, calling out "¡Hola!" and "¡Buenas dias!" He ran up the slight incline to the Church of Guadalupe, but was surprised to find that he was having some trouble breathing. It didn't matter. He was just happy to be back. He stopped, caught his breath, and looked up at the crown atop the bell tower. Supported by a circle of angels, it turned golden in the late afternoon sunlight. Looking down at the Pacific, he took a deep breath and let it out. How peaceful he was beginning to feel! He walked down to the beach, stood there for a few minutes, and then took off his shoes and socks. The sand felt good under his feet. As he walked toward the water, Jack stared at the sun that hung in the sky like a slowly whirling ball of fire. Suddenly he became aware that, except for the sshh of the waves and the sound of his own breathing, the town was silent and empty. It made him uneasy. Then he sensed someone behind him and turning came face to face with the angel who smiled sweetly and put out his hand.

A.I.D.S (Africa Is Dying Swiftly)

Ghariokwu Lemi

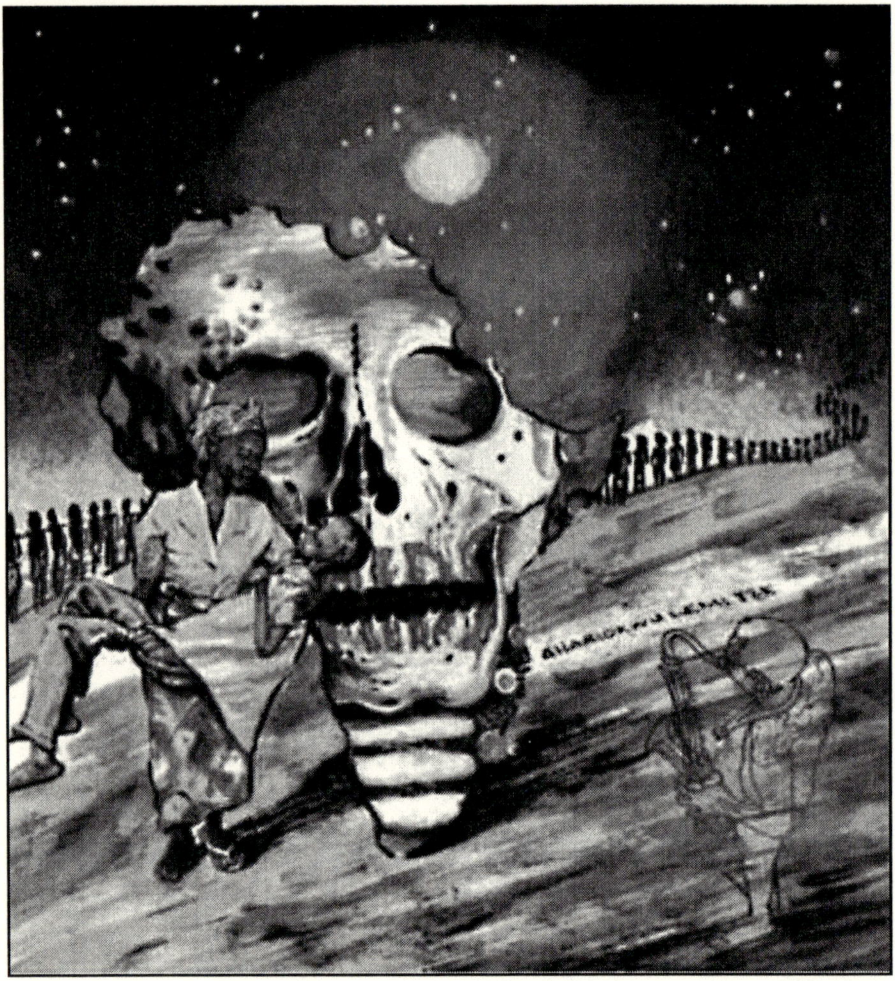

diagnosis

Raymond Berry

i recall unuttered words and urges
i thought would open unused life
but instead conceived a wound

maybe it was inescapable
sacrificing safeness for sensation
now mortality wants answers

this thing does not judge
called to do what is asked.
create shadows that move when i am still

Split Personality

Kevin McLellan

i. Ugly Bouquet

The tulip wanted to be the rose
and the rose wanted to be the tulip

until both realized that as each other
they would still be cut; and then

they both wanted to be a raven
on the highest branch until they

realized that they would not
bring beauty to tables.

ii. Jugular

The foreign shapes inside

my blood: on the dizzying
track, a circle becomes

lightheaded: loses track of

time. My neck is in front
of who I am becoming or

rather what I have become:
circulation dictates the how:

the how to not strain.

iii. Beautiful Utensils

My veins are now outside my neck. The flying
white-necked raven with beak and talons. The feeling
to skin after a warm shower on a warm day; and
breeze through an open window blows. Yet, regret
doesn't exist here. Nor does

ice cream or spoons or the hands of others.

Faith of My Own

Keith R. Green

Outside of fertilizing the seed that would become me, my father's role in my life is of no real significance. Having been together for several years without marrying, he and my mother parted ways very shortly after I was born. From then on, I'd only see him during the infrequent occasions that he allowed himself to be bothered.

When I was about four years old, my mother married a man who turned out to be cruel. I can recall numerous occasions where verbal and physical interactions between us became intense enough to convince me that he outright hated me, for reasons about which I am still not clear. There is one thing that I'm certain of though, and it's those negative relationships would serve as precursors to what I would experience in relationships with other men.

Roy was 30 when I met him, and I was but an impressionable and helplessly naïve 19-year-old tenderoni. Okay...maybe not so naïve, but most certainly impressionable, and unquestionably starving for the attention of an older male figure.

He caught my eye as he was standing incognito in a dark corner at the Jeffrey Pub, Chicago's longest operating gay bar. Underneath a hoodie and the brim of an all black Chicago White Sox cap, his solid five-foot-ten athletic build and woogie-boy demeanor set him apart from the abundance of old "queens" who typically frequented the bar. Of course I wasn't old enough to be in there, but I'd been a regular since I was 17. Harvey the doorman was relentlessly trying to have me and my crew of friends, so gaining access was never an issue.

I peeped Roy watching me while I was out on the dance floor, getting my life to a remix of the latest Janet Jackson banger. Once I was certain that it was me who he was checking for, I decided I'd heat things up a bit and give him a show. I've always loved to dance, and Janet's music is notorious for bringing out my suppressed stripper fantasies. Grinding and gyrating seductively to the track's throbbing baseline, I allowed my body language to express to Roy exactly what I was thinking about doing to him, or what I wanted him to do to me. He got the message, and soon signaled for me to come over and talk to him.

I can't recall the exact nature of our conversation, but I do know that I was deeply engaged in whatever it was. He was intelligent, in a very masculine, street-smart kind of way. His lips were longingly kissable, and his eyes were mesmerizing.

After a couple of drinks we realized that we'd lost track of time. We'd been sitting across from the bar talking as if we were the only two people there for just long enough to make it a reality. It was closing time and, as we agreed to exchange numbers and hook up again soon, I realized that my ride had somehow managed to leave without me. When he offered to take me home, I knew instantly that I was in for a long night.

What I couldn't have imagined though, was that that fateful night would turn into days, and those days into years — four years, to be exact. I also couldn't have predicted, but would soon find out, that he was married and that he served as a minister at a church on Chicago's Westside. And, although I had disclosed my HIV status to him very early on in our courtship, I wouldn't learn that he too was HIV positive until we'd been seeing each other for nearly a year. As layered as the situation quickly became, however, I found myself so helplessly entangled inside of this man's web that there was no walking away. If there were a cure for him, I didn't want it. I was in love.

Although I was intrigued by everything that I was learning about him, it was the revelation of his HIV status that knocked me off my square. Why hadn't he told me when I told him? Did his wife know? Was she positive too? What about their daughter? I shot off a boatload of questions at him, the answers to which I soon realized I was completely unprepared for.

He explained to me that he had been living with HIV for more than seven years, and that his wife did in fact know. She was negative, he told me, and so was their child. He said that he'd led her to believe that he'd become infected from an accident involving a needle-stick, which happened while he was working at a local hospital. She had no knowledge of his sexual rendezvous with other men.

(Obviously I wasn't the only person to succumb to the magical spell of this man!)

By both of their accounts (I would eventually become close enough with her that she would ask me to be the godfather of their second child), when their pastor married them he'd prayed that their serodiscordant status would not be a barrier in their relationship, and that Shawnette would remain uninfected. Through Roy's unwavering faith, or some random miracle, God had answered that prayer.

I was in complete and utter awe as I tried to process all that I was being told. When I was first diagnosed with HIV in the mid-nineties, I was certain that I was living on borrowed time. It was, after all, a couple of years before the advent of protease inhibitors and the resulting "Lazarus effect" that many people who were dying of AIDS experienced by taking them. At 17 years old, I was certain that I'd never live to see 25, although I'd heard a little voice within me whispering otherwise. And now, standing before me was this beautiful specimen of a man who refused to accept the fatality of AIDS, and as a result seemed to be evading such an untimely death. He was living an alternative reality that was simply based on his faith. I was wondering if I could somehow experience the same.

I latched on to Roy like a lost puppy to the first lowly human to offer him refuge. I became a sponge, sopping up any and all information that I could about this "great faith" that seemed to be a lifestyle for him rather than some abstract ideal. When I asked him how I might go about acquiring such faith, he told me that it was as simple as learning to trust and believe in God. He believed beyond a shadow of a doubt that God had healed his body of HIV and blindly trusted that everything would work out for him. As a result, he refused to take medications because, in his mind, to do so would constitute a lack of genuine faith. He advised me that if I really wanted to be healed, I had to exercise faith of that same magnitude. And so, without hesitation, I completely stopped taking the drugs that had been prescribed to me.

...

For the next six years, I would live "HIV-med" free. Roy's inability to completely and openly commit to another man caused our relationship to slowly wither away. We remained friends, but as I matured I became less and less tolerant of living inside of a closet with him. I needed to be free to explore the other rooms in the house.

I continued to trust and believe in God, however, as my faith and understanding of Him grew considerably with time. I'd begun to attend church with Roy while we were together, but would eventually leave that church to branch out on my own. I'd learned so much from him that in my new church home I was soon asked to assist with teaching Sunday School and, eventually, to join the Junior Deacon's Board. Things were going well for me because of my newly found faith, and then it was tested.

HIV began to take its devastating toll on my body. My six foot four inch frame, which averaged around 190 pounds was slowly reduced to a mere 144 pounds. My t-cell count dropped to 30 at 6 percent, and my viral load shot up well above a million. Doctors told me to get my affairs in order because it looked as though I wouldn't be around for more than a year.

I began to question whether I truly possessed the faith that was necessary for overcoming this HIV demon. Or was I living more off the faith of others than I cared to acknowledge?

Time would reveal that both notions were true to some extent. My faith was fledgling and had not been tested up until that point. I am sure that there were moments when Roy's incredible faith had also been tried, but the key to his success had been to never stop believing, no matter how bad things appeared to be. I had learned the basics of having great faith from him, and it was now time for me to practice the skills for myself.

apocrypha
jamila woods

"Black women are an endangered species"
—HIV activist Suzanna Engo

I could tell you how little girls grow up
grow girls little how you tell

I could speak in backwards words
back in speak could I
cause we can't speak of this
forwards

her lips are tied in his
like shoelaces in fingers before she learned how
he doubledutched them into bows
worthy of little girls' foreheads on Sundays
said, it's safer that way
loose laces don't mix with fast paces
wouldn't want you to trip n ruin how pretty your face is-

and her lips are tied like this
even lying on mattresses
lightly finger painting canvasses
but he craves masterpieces
with bigger brush strokes—

simon says go
and he asks nicely

but she knows what simon says goes
and she's only saying no with her eyes
a language he can't recognize

more ancient than ABCs but
he's too busy writing Latin stems
against her hem
with tongue-inked pen
she's staring at the ceiling
tyring to keep from screaming
singing soft songs in her head like

red rover red rover came over
came rover red rover red
shoulda listened to what mama said
sweaty hands don't do no good at
keeping out strangers

who come in without wiping their feet at the door
they don't leave even after you've fed them
everything you've got
they won't leave
until you do
you til un leave won't they
we can't speak of this

orange canisters with white plastic lids
doctors feed her this
peer at her with pity eyes
like what a *shame* you is
can't even save yourself from your own sins

miss mary mack
all colored black
with purple bruises
all down her back

and her body don't belong to her anymore
she wonders if it *ever* did
ever it if wonders she

these impolite guests
play hide go seek
in tiny hallways beneath her skin
they always win
and she stays poppin pills tryna feel
normal again

I could tell you how little girls grow up
grow girls little how you tell
I could speak in backwards words
back in speak could I

cause we can't speak of this forwards
we can't speak of this with words—

just red loop ribbons on shirts
days made to remind us to remember
newscasts stats and numbers
but what she's lost can't be measured
and we can't speak of this for *words*

can't ever explain

A Long Ride To Nowhere

Geoffrey D. Holman AKA Priest

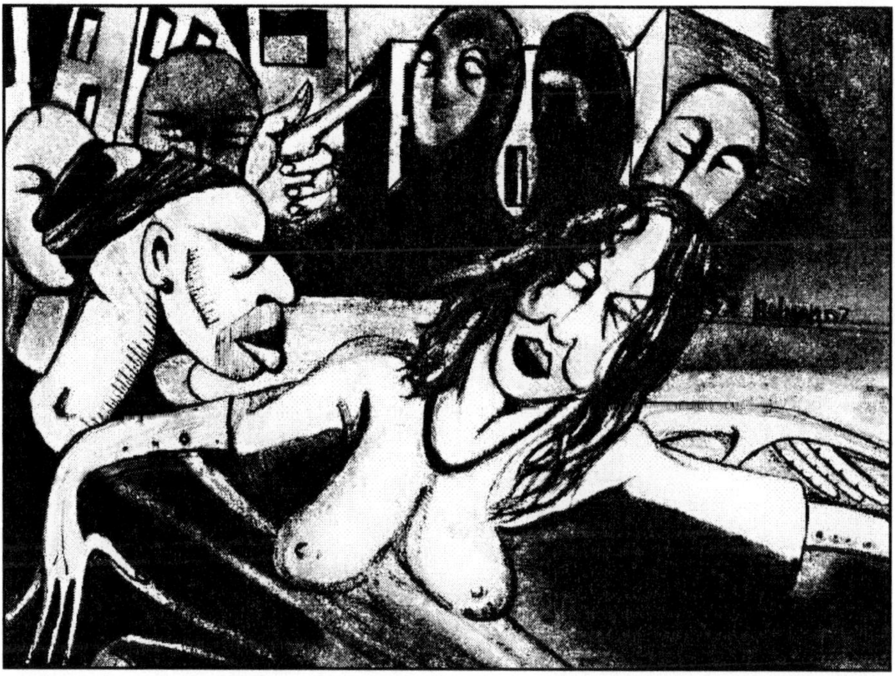

Mouth Pebble

Chloe' Yelena Miller

Italia

(Male) gray veins navigate the surface, thumbnail sized
(white as the paint stains on his overalls) pebble, baked,
centered between the cod's
hair-thick bones *(your hand*
on his stomach until morning).

You dislodge it with your fork and knife,
(his mother didn't know she was feeding his lover)
never touching the food with your bus-pole-dirty fingers
(you are discreet).

Digested once, it added weight to the market scale
(he told you your hair was too feminine).

Too large to hide behind your teeth,
(he wouldn't kiss you buona notte)
under your tongue
(he infected you).

Antibodies

Shanna Germain

At twenty, I started working the HIV
ward, midnight to morning. Left my husband
sleeping, mouth-open to the air, to
drive through the dark body of the city.

Every shift, the warning about infections.
Me sliding on booties, disposable
gown and gloves. Even through the mask,
you could smell decay, the way viruses

swept through bodies. I did what was needed:
held hands through double-gloves, took blood
or confessions when I could, told off-white lies
to thin cracked lips that knew the truth.

Once, a year or so into it, I stuck
myself, pointed red end of an IV needle
left in a lab coat pocket. So small a thing
it almost didn't hurt going in, only

leaving, small pop and smear of two bloods mingled.
I put the wound to my mouth and sucked before
I thought. Fear rising, rinsed my tongue with soap,
spit someone's dark blood into the white scrub sink,

then gave my own blood to one of the other nurses
to be tested. At dawn, I roused my husband awake
with my newly tainted tongue, let him slide bare
into me, as though nothing was between us.

I tell this all like it was an accident:
someone else's lab coat, a needle forgotten
in a white pocket, three seconds of married
passion so strong my lips did not say, at risk.

But no. This was after I caught the cliché
of my life: his red scrawl across receipts hidden
in a desk drawer, the smell of lilacs in
his sleeves, the cleaving across the bedsides.

The things we do in fear are the things we don't
say. Hidden and rampant as a hotel room stay
on a credit card, or a string of genes
in a coat of protein, destined to repeat.

How to Be Promiscuous in an Epidemic

Viet Lê

We seek refuge in the Buddha, the dharma, the sangha.
—Tibetan prayer

I.

Driving to the 24 hour Korean tofu joint, on 6th
through the dimlit homes, tall shadows
past Wilshire, our conversation curving, like the asphalt:
you research in psychology-poverty
and African American communities; Tibetan Buddhism.

Tibetan Buddhism allows me to think of mortality,
including my own . . .

. . . I am positive, you said

and it is something I try to imagine
how my world would change-unyielding, dimlit like the row of houses, a blur
and swerve-
but cannot

and what I wanted to say in response:
Buddhism is about mortality, the ever present
we could die at any moment

instead of my awkwardness, *it is about awareness, being present,*
changing the topic

but what to say?
That I am afraid that it may be me too, soon.
And how will that change things,
my love, oh stranger, my friend?

What half-life waits us, the kitchen clock, the tall glass of water?

The breach the gap
my body's—
            I am afraid, and cannot get beyond that.

II.

I am tired of always asking eye to eye
tired of second guessing their answers.
Last time

I didn't want to know, didn't care to know.

Tired of that tired look
in your eye, Ron, Michael, Douglas, Rick, Patrick,
Anthony, Tommy, Jason... your generic names,
names I've forgotten, armies
of the dead and living.
I am sick

of thinking, *this is the last time I may see you.*

Crossing that invisible line

the hollow of your cheeks,

what will I look like,
paler, skinnier than now?

Will I recognize myself in you?

What refuge is there?

Contraction

Chanell Ruth

It is not your death sentence but it is
You can give it to someone you love, but you shouldn't
They said it wouldn't become our disease, but it did
You could do it again, but you wouldn't

You could have prevented it, but you didn't
Thought he/she wasn't infected, but she/he was
They said it was a *gay thing*, but it isn't
It doesn't have to kill you but it does

Tried to stop it but we couldn't
Could cease to love, but we can't
Say you have been careful, but you haven't
Could choose to stop living but you shan't

Could tell the world our story, but we won't
Need to take responsibility, but we don't

A Secret Code

Lamont Steptoe

In memory of Essex Hemphill & Joseph F. Beam

In the Age of AIDS to be tested is a duty. The lapse of time between knowing and not knowing is a quagmire of emotion. What if I am positive? This followed immediately by an assertion, "I can't possibly be positive! I was always atop. I never swallowed anything. I never had a discharge in the rectum!" But something brings you to the public health center crowded like a supermarket, crowded like an army depot with recruits, crowded like an unemployment office, crowded like a welfare office.

All the walls papered with warnings. Red letters giving the odds, citing the risks. In numerous places the message — THERE IS NO CURE FOR AIDS! And here you are among the ones who took a chance, followed a blind instinct, gave into a loneliness or lust powerful enough to cause you to cast caution to the wind.

Still it's like a dream. You don't feel sick. You don't feel doomed. You have plans enough to fill up 80+ years, yet just last week you memorialized a Black poet like yourself, although younger. Two months ago, he was alive and now he's memory...history...an ancestor. Will you follow in his footsteps, die the painful, techno-death he died? You are here to find out. Some voice inside cries out to God. "I get it now! Spare me this time and I won't open myself to such risk again! Spare me God! There's all the writing to be done. There's the years with my child. There's the struggle with my people for freedom. Spare me God! Let me be HERE not OVER THERE! Don't let this be the beginning of my exit from the world! Don't let this public impersonal factory be the gateway to doom for me! Why am I here? Why am I not ensconced in a secure relationship that fulfills my desires, keeps me tied to one person who desires only me? Why did I let my emotions herd me from bath house to bar to theaters hot with the passion of sex and lust?

Now that I have heard these things, now that I have witnessed men worshipping men, swallowing hot semen or humping unprotected asses for a moment of ecstasy, now that I have heard, smelled and witnessed such passion, will I be allowed to escape, be allowed to live to tell the tale of the dead or am I fated to die in the telling, shrinking like a Dracula caught in sunlight? Such lovely faces shining in the dark, eyes reflecting cinematic images upside down and backwards, as they scan the darkness for a partner. Who are these death angels locked in a dance of desire? Boys and men like me, fathers and sons, uncles and grandparents, all lonely for love. Young men, middle aged men, old men, down on their knees, hungry for big swollen cocks in the mouth, in the ass or hungry to lick the fruit of the anus — tongue it like a pomegranate, digging deeper and deeper with tongue, spearing that sensitive mouth that drives its recipient to ecstasy, to ejaculation, forgetting everything but the act. Forgetting the danger, forgetting the quagmire of emotions, that haunt the weeks following the act risking all for a Moment, a FLEETING MOMENT, gone even as it comes!

435, 620, 730, 628, the numbers called out, shouted out like someone must call them out from the other side of life and we wait for OUR NUMBER to be called. It's like this, just like this! We HEAR OUR NUMBER, we rise and follow the caller trembling, uncertain of WHERE WE ARE GOING, how soon we will arrive. We enter a strange room, greeted by a stranger, who will bleed us, capture our blood in a glass tube, send it out to other strangers, who will judge us as clean or unclean. Other strangers, who will tell us if we are to live or DIE! But not immediately, no, we must WAIT and PRAY. We consider EVERYTHING we have done up to this moment. We must consider everything we would like to do beyond this moment as well. We have two weeks to ponder our fate. Will the chips fall on the red or the black? Will we believe it if our number comes up? Will we CRY? SCREAM? RUN? DANCE? SHOUT? BREAK SOMETHING? OR JUST CRUMPLE LIKE A RAG DOLL?

Our Momma's birthed us for this ending? Birthed us to die of a plague? Birthed us to be a quilted name, a victim of horror pounding on death's door?

The blood is drawn. One turns away as it rushes into the tube with its secrets. Why couldn't the virus make it sparkle, or turn yellow or even have barber stripes just so we would know instantly? The hole in the artery is plugged with cotton, bandaged. We are sent away with our secret code, sent away into the streets, back to lovers, children, family, and fellow workers. We are sent away to ponder the meaning of life. Leaving, we scan the faces in the lobby of the public health center. How many are the living dead? Are YOU one of them? Common faces, young faces. So many BLACKS! So many BROWNS! ALL WANTING TO KNOW THEIR SENTENCE! But what was their CRIME? Needing LOVE? Needing human companionship? Needing to be needed? In the 90s and now the 21st century, it's a crime to be needed. It's a crime to be loved. The sentence: death! Someone doesn't want so many Blacks, Browns, so many Gays, needing to be needed. Someone doesn't want so many Blacks, Browns, so many Gays, needing to be needed. Someone doesn't want so many Blacks, Browns, Gays loving each other. Young men, virile, muscular, beautiful chests, bubble buttocks, Grecian calves, a poet's lips and eyes-all doomed. Women are also here to find out after having found out their men were on the DL (downlow), exposing them to the virus with unprotected sex. The lobby filled with life is also filled with death. Things moving so fast it's not years that count anymore, it's not months or even weeks, it's minutes and seconds-in this age. We tell our years on earth in minutes. I'm seven thousand minutes old. I'm sixteen thousand minutes old. I'm forty thousand minutes old. I'm five hundred and thirty five thousand six hundred seconds old. I'm ten million seven hundred and twelve thousand seconds old. I'm sixteen million sixty eight thousand seconds old...we say goodbye to our friends as if they are called away to war because indeed, they have been and will be called away to war. Armed only with love, our friends are falling, casualties of an invisible enemy, a master of guerilla warfare. Thousands even millions are dying but WHO IS KILLING THEM? The body count mounts and mounts and mounts and we cannot find the enemies' tracks. The enemy has no face, no address, and no country. Or is the enemy our neighbor in the suit and tie and lab coat? Armed only with LOVE, we die like millions of Christs mumbling...FATHER FORGIVE THEM THEY KNOW WHAT THEY DO!

Georgie Kissed A Boy

Toni Asante Lightfoot

Georgie was a gorgeous boy.
So fine I knew I wasn't like my cousin.
She liked girls. I liked Georgie.

The neighborhood held him close.
He loved us all as we were.
We loved him for all he wasn't.
Georgie wasn't like us.

Georgie remembered our birthdays,
our favorite colors, the things
you shouldn't say to us.
Georgie grew up opposite from the man

who aided in his death. Jacob's neighborhood
still doesn't know his life
was filled with a love they would've
beaten him to death for living.

Jacob met Georgie at a voguer's ball.
Georgie was the belle he always was.
Jacob stood strong recklessly eyeballing
the confident beauty.

Jacob drove a mustang a lie like a pimp drives
a corner — relentlessly menacing but with style.
Everyone wanted to believe his fabulousness

as it flew down the street to the stop sign.
Jacob spent his short time in the closet
scared, angry, and abused.
Didn't know the men he hid with
held deadly secrets under their skin.

It was the '90s. Before we knew
how Black skin turns pallid
when invaded by killer cells.

Georgie lived for love. Jacob lived
longer for Georgie's love. Jacob paid
for his closet space with their lives.

When Georgie laid to rest
folks from the neighborhood
showed up with flowers and real
tears because Georgie wasn't like us.

When Jacob took his final ride
we were there too. Georgie made us
better.

Hi My Name is Julia

Mila Rozen

My name is Julia and all my life I've been thinking of becoming a model. I finally took the plunge when I was 19. There were a few agencies in my city and I decided to visit them all. Frankly, I was fed up with the state of my life at this moment in time. I had an ambition.

From an early age my mother and I were victims of abuse by my father. Before I was born, my father forced my mum to have three abortions, and when she finally decided to keep her fourth child, which was me, dad had abandoned us for America. That is why I am the only child.

He never sent us any alimony or financial support, so life was tough. My mother had to do demeaning part-time jobs in the evening on top of her full-time job as a lab assistant in a hospital just to make ends meet.

My dad returned to us ten years after he left and blamed us for all his failings, including not being able to achieve his lifelong ambition of becoming an architect and having to settle for a job as a draughtsman. He fared no better in New York, working in construction and blaming us for that as well.

All he achieved in the U.S. was to make enough money to buy a two-bedroom flat on a council block and a new car. He also managed to persuade my mother to move back with him, which my mum agreed because life was so hard being a single parent in Poland. He goes drinking every day with his "so-called" friends, who are also alcoholics, and continues to use mum and I as punching bags. His plan for me was to follow his ambition to become an architect. But when I failed my entrance exams, he beat me up.

I thought my life was looking up when I met my boyfriend, but he promptly dumped me when he was accepted into a university. His father was wealthy, and my chance to marry into a good family passed me by.

Modeling seemed like my only way out. I would travel, meet new people, make money and spend money. The whole of Warsaw would envy me, and that is the way

I dreamt things should be. My mother and I deserved it after all we had been through. It has often been said that I am beautiful, charismatic and photogenic. My hair colour was dark brown, but I dyed it blond and my pitch black eyes were oval shaped. I am only five feet, seven inches tall, which may not be enough for the catwalk, but becoming a photographic model could suit me best.

I dialed the number of the agency my friend recommended and was asked to come in for an interview. I subsequently met a woman in her forties, who introduced herself as Grazyna. She was really pleasant to me, almost as nice as my mother. We would always meet in the nicest places in Warsaw. Grazyna took an instant liking to me and suggested that I would make a perfect model and make a great success of it.

Every time we met, she tried to persuade me to allow her to represent me, by explaining the real lives of models. It sounded like heaven to me. She really made me think I could inhabit that special peak of fame reserved only for a chosen few: Kate Moss, Naomi Campbell and even Carla Bruni. Grazyna promised she would open doors for me, behind which there would be an Aladdin's cave of treasures. She went on to explain that one had to start somewhere.

"Look at yourself, at your clothes. You will never win any casting unless you are well presented. I will fund this initial transformation and you would pay me back when you start to earn money," she said.

Grazyna spent a good few thousand Zloty on Fendi, Versace and Gucci bags and shoes — the best of Haut Couture; the only way to start, in her opinion. I hesitated a little but I had begun to trust her. Why would she spend all this money if she did not believe in me? I was nobody, didn't have enough money to get to Paris or Milan or rent a flat. I was broke. How was I going to get to castings? How many "go-sees" would I attend before I got my first assignment? I had to trust her. (It was only a couple years later that I realised those bags were fakes).

Grazyna sent me to Monaco, which did not sound too bad. I was meant to be a hostess but when I got there I realised that we had to do sex for money. With no language, no money to go back, I had no choice but to follow the rest of girls. My first client was around 70 years old and bald and he knew I had never done it before so his desire was to have sex without a condom. I agreed, besides I was not in a position to argue. I didn't feel anything either. Frankly, when I think about it now, someone must have spiked my drink, otherwise how on earth could four men have fucked me on my first night? The more I thought about what happened, the more crap I felt about myself. Next day I called up Grazyna and complained that she did not inform me about the "job" in detail.

"Naomi Campbell, Cindy Crawford stripped for money," she responded. "Nobody seems to see anything wrong in it. Madonna worked in sex-shops, and today she is a millionaire. Different models started their careers in different ways. You've got to make sacrifices in order to achieve something in life. This is show business and not a convent. Girls have to sleep with bookers, photographers, agency owners. I told you exactly what to do. Before you went there, I took you to Paris and spent $700 on you. Don't waste my time and money. The prince is there somewhere and you have to be nice to him. If he wants to be with you, you have to do it. Who did you think you are, princess?"

"But we did not discuss sleeping for money before I came here?"

"Wouldn't you sleep with a prince, who would care for you and would be lovely to you? Stop talking crap. You don't have to sleep with him every day, but it's enough if you agree you will be with him. To have such a man as a friend is a privilege, an honour. You have to change your mind for your own good."

Grazyna went on a tangent.

I don't know what prince she was talking about because no royalty ever came by where I was working. I decided to do sex for money only once in my lifetime. Who knows, maybe she was right, and my next client could even be a prince.

After a week or so, I was paid my first salary and it gave me a feel good factor. I put out all the dollar notes in front of me like Tarot cards. The future was rosy and all the cards meant fortune. As soon as I make enough money, I thought, *I will look for modeling job.*

I had to learn how to put up with someone's dick that smelled like a dairy factory hit by atomic mushroom or how to have sex with three guys on Viagra at the same time, which was exhausting. Over time my new job became a tolerable pain. Some of the girls became my good friends. We compensated our hardships with treating ourselves to certain pleasurable pursuits such as shopping, beauty spas and holidays. In the end we had so much in common. Most of us had cruel fathers, no fathers or alcoholic fathers and no support from them. We had to take care of ourselves. We worked mainly in London, Milan and Paris. But the Arabs paid the most, so we frequently visited Saudi Arabia, the United Arab Emirates and Lebanon. Saudi Arabia was a top secret project as we flew in on a private plane, all wrapped up in black clothes that Arab women usually wear. All I saw was a brothel, as I was not allowed to go out. Girls were Eastern European, English, Italian and French — all beautiful and blond.

I really wanted my friends in Poland to think that I succeeded in life, so I told them I travelled to Saudi Arabia to do make-up shows and that I dated a prince. They believed me. In fact all those silly girls I met in bars believed that my father was a professor in Architecture and my mum was a doctor. My new boyfriend Borys (who is my current partner) wasn't so naïve though. I met him at a Miss of Poland event and over time I realised his life wasn't any better either. He dropped out of law school and was selling fake watches. Soon afterwards, I found myself supporting him financially. I needed him and he needed me. In the end we were so similar. His father left him when he was a child too.

My father started to cause problems again. He must have watched a program on TV about European prostitutes working in Arab countries and he started to call me a prostitute, beating me and mum again. I love my mum very much and when I make a lot of money, I promise I will buy a house for me and her to move into. Mum's sister has schizophrenia and I recently gave her a job as a cleaner at my boyfriend's flat, where I moved in recently and for which I had been paying anyway.

I have to support them all but I am tired of it. I don't want to work for my agent Grazyna either as she takes half my salary. I want to go independent and have girls working for me. Being advised by my boyfriend, I decide to offer it to one of my friends, Ola. They all seemed to know my secret anyway; they are not as stupid as I thought. Someone called up my parent's house the other day and left a message

"Dear Madam and Sir, you daughter is a whore." It took me a lot of effort to change my parent's number. I hate them all, besides Coco and Irenka who have been the only loyal and real friends to me all those years.

I meet up with Ola. She is good looking and could be a model. She is a bit surprised to hear me saying "I am a prostitute" but when I asked her if she knew, she responded that she suspected it. Well, it is my fault. I shouldn't have said I travelled to Saudi, anywhere else in the world but Saudi. Ola has a boyfriend and said she is not interested in my offer. We are different at the end of the day. Her father never beat her mum or called her a whore, but he once gave me a lift, and from the way he looked at me I knew he would like to fuck me, as if all those men had a sort of sixth sense.

Ola said she does not have to sleep with a millionaire for money because she could easily marry one. She mentioned the book she is writing so I changed the topic. I hate her for having a decent life and dreams. In fact the only reason I met with her is because I enjoy hating her. She is pathetic.

"How risky is it to catch HIV in that job?" Ola asked.

"There are more chances for you to get a cold than HIV." I cut her short.

"Well of course there are. If you said I am more likely to win a lottery than HIV I would consider it," she laughed.

I realised what I just said was utterly stupid, but I am just repeating something someone once said about HIV without thinking much about it. It actually sounds as stupid as believing that fucking a little child would cure you of AIDS in parts of Africa.

Frankly, I don't even want to think about that risk. I slept with at least 50 men without using a condom. If I started thinking about the probabilities, permutations, the likelihood of getting infected with AIDS, I would go nuts like my auntie. I was negative the last time I was tested two years ago. I still ended up with a tough HPV virus.

I found out recently that my Italian friend Erica got HIV. She confessed it to her best friend Silvio and everyone knows about it now. I checked her Facebook and instead of profile picture she put an animated painting of cute skulls on a pink background. Erica keeps popping back in my mind. I am wondering how she is doing now? Was she infecting clients, who would unconsciously infect other prostitutes or their wives?

I wanted to get on with my life. But it was so difficult. I worried all the time that someone would find out about my past and ask questions. I really don't need to have HIV on my mind. I have had enough of herpes, gonorrhea and syphilis. You name it, I had it and have been on some sort of medication since it all started. But I hold on to that day me and Erica ended up in a triangle with a client...was she already infected? When was it? She pretended to be my friend only to have lesbian sex, which I did not enjoy. When exactly was the last time I had a HIV test? Oh my fucking God, it really hit me like a hammer, it felt like someone is putting a gun to my head. What are the chances for me to be positive? Positive, negative, positive, negative, my head was spinning.

I felt so lonely. There was no one I could discuss this with. My boyfriend would hit me and call me the worst possible names. If he left me, I would be on my own again. He is the only person I am totally honest with, besides my beloved friends Coco and Irenka. How much would I pay for them to be real and not just a product of my imaginative childhood, when I had no sisters to talk to, just dolls?

"We are your friends no matter what" Coco smiled.

"Leave me!" I cry tormented "Stop following me! You know nothing about real life."

Waiting List

Marguerite L. Harrold

I no longer scan the list before hand
Most names I don't recognize anyway
Lots of new people
Lots of men now
Straight ones too
I guess this means things have really gotten bad
Straight men are always the last to follow trends
Always the last to worry

Please Take A Ticket

Richard Sawdon Smith

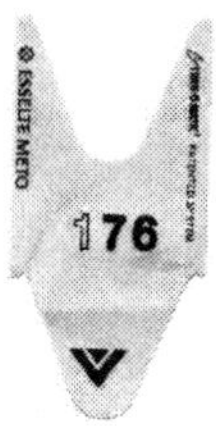

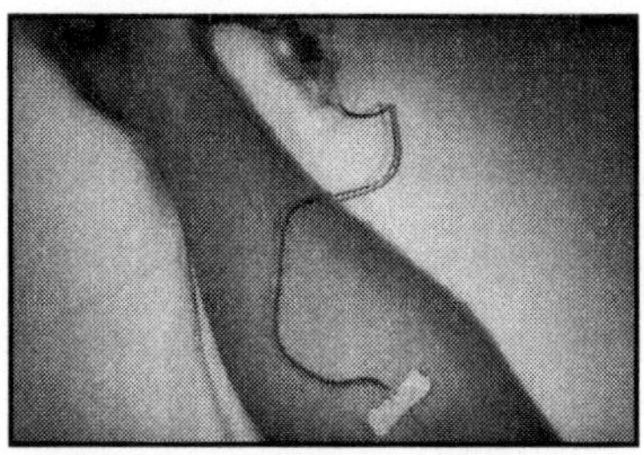

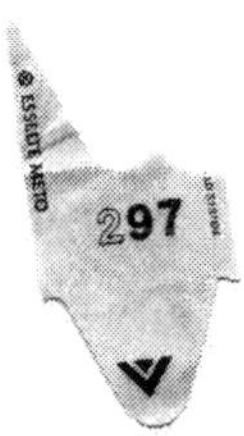

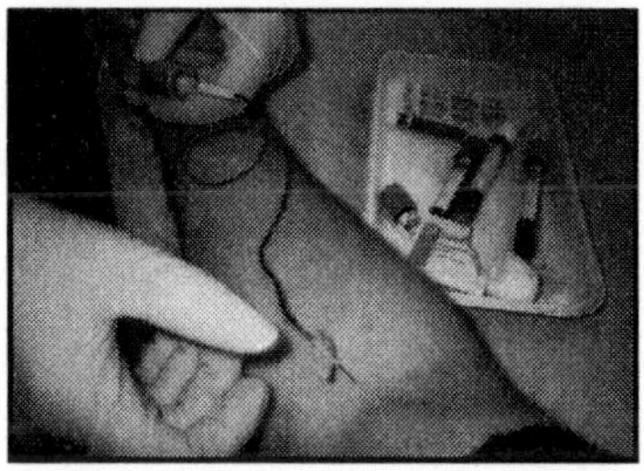

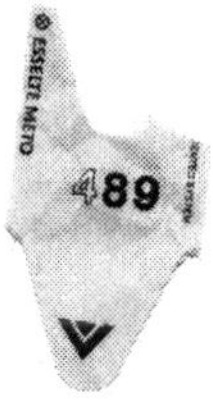

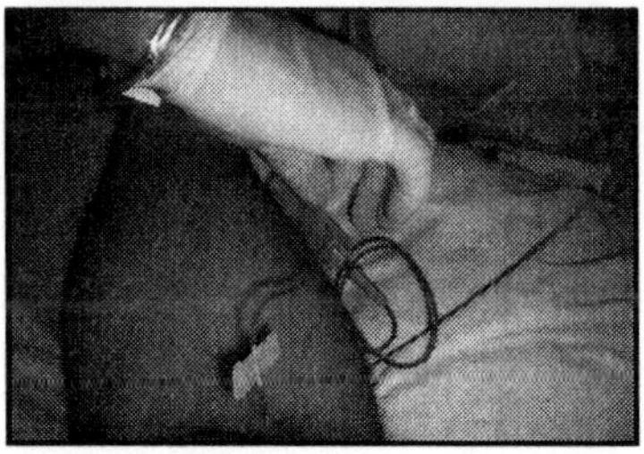

The Early Bird gets the John

Derrick Harriell

Madeline wipes fog off the tattered mirror,
fixing eyes on fresh lines forming across her forehead.
She fumbles through purse for mascara and foundation,
leaves mace buried beneath a rubbish of forsaken innocence.
For a slight moment, she recalls the reflection before prom,
the pressed hair and vibrant skin, the happy eyes
and virgin lips. On that day, a popular junior waited downstairs.
Today, a crumpled senior waits in the other room.
He wants to feel the fire one last time,
to tell her she's beautiful before she walks away.

Secret

Michael Broder

Remember when walks on the beach
Led to trysts in the cool sand beneath the boardwalk?

Disease then crept through your body,
but you kept it at bay with a churning engine of desire.

Now you wash the virus away
like silt through a hollow drainpipe,

and this life now is the better life, but oh,
how the cool sand calls.

Francine Francis (age 13)
Red Hook Housing Projects, Brooklyn, NY

Tony Medina

Dear Santa,

I'm writing you because I'm sad.
My older sister got AIDS from a needle
when she used to do drugs.
I can't stand to see her suffer.
She is always in so much pain.
My mother had to take off from
work to take care of her because
she's always either sick in the bed
with diarhea and numonia or
going to the hospital because she
don't eat or could hardly breathe.

My mother almost got fired from her
job because she took so many days
off from work to take care of her.
Sometimes I leave school early
so I could be there to help
her clean up or go to the bathroom.
I try to cook things she could eat
without getting tired or throwing up
all the time like she does.

What I'm askin for is nothing for
me but for my sister and mother.
We need money to be able to take
her to a better hospital cause
the one she go to is too
dirty and crowded and it take
too long for the doctor to help.
Plus the medicine is too much
money and my mother could
hardly afford it.

If you send the money
to help us, I promise
when I get out of school
and get a job we'll pay you
back.

The Two Genevas

Gwendolyn A. Mitchell

I. Geneva one.

I am not afraid to tell his/my story
a mother's love/a sacrifice
the living through storm, survival, loss and memory.
What else do I have to do
except save another woman from this pain of silence?
I'm an old woman now
and have more yesterdays than tomorrows.
I no longer lose sleep with questions,
I am answer, living proof of
what you don't know can kill.

II. Geneva two.

You watched me raise my children
raised you too—in and out of my house on any given day
did not know what secrets to keep, what to tell.
Even now, we don't have conversations beyond cordialities.

All my life I've been fighting battles for schools,
for children, neighborhoods,
for freedom from questions,
but my activist spirit
is silenced
not knowing how to speak a
living litany
of words
I forget. For what am I thankful?

III. Geneva one.

He didn't try to be anyone else.
That's why they all loved him-
every Sunday the disciplined, controlled,
masterful musician,
not wanting justification,
not needing excuse,
but seeking audience with God.

IV. Geneva two.

I'd like to tell you
that it didn't make a difference
that it didn't bother me
to limit our conversations around his father
who would pass the phone after grunting a
greeting, then leave the room;
that at Christmas and New Years there
would always be old schoolmates present—
women I knew from yearbook pictures—invited
just to keep up appearances.
I'd like to tell you
it didn't make a difference.

V. Genevas together.

We, in our separate grief,
in our knowing that
we were not silent types, were not meant to hold tongues,
share this celebration of sons,
this defiance, this quiet beauty of what was never ours to keep
We, two women of gardens, music and safe crossing over deep waters,
search each other's hearts for understanding.

Blouse and Skirt

Kwame Dawes

So the other day, I'm walking through Edgewater
to go look for my sister, and I'm minding
my own business. It hot, but hot is not
sickness, and hot is better than cold, and
I know how to walk easy and stay cool;
so I am walking and minding my own business,
and maybe it was the way I slow it down—
true the heat make me move kinda
sweet, and it's only skirt I wear
these days after I realize that too much
heat up your leg can steam up
your body and my business need breeze—
and I know how to work a good
pleat skirt; so even in my flat shoes,
and even with my pick-picky head,
looking like nobody don't touch
it with money for months, I can
make a man stop what he is doing,
look twice, maybe more, cause Jamaican
man can't help themselves, cause
its pure browning pussy they want.
And that is just what happen that day.
This man drive up and blow horn
and start sweet talk me, tell me
what he can do to me, how he can
make me feel so good I will forget
my own name; I kiss my teeth

and keep on walking, and he following
even though all kind of car blowing
and cussing him for holding up
the traffic. When I look I see
he is a good looking man, but same
time I tell him, "Man, you don't want
this pumpum, baby, trust me." But him
go on and go on till I have to say
to him, "Massa, me have AIDS,
you want dead?" And me? — a woman
who don't care — is sorry I sorry
for this fool with his nice car,
good teeth, pretty face and nice hair.
"No problem," him say. "AIDS
is nothing to me." No lie. Just so
he say it to my face, so I ask him,
"Massa, you don't know trouble?"
And I go on walking, especially when
I see the big fat ring on him finger.
Yet when I see that this is a fool,
this is a careless Ethiopian, I think
to myself, you know how easy and sweet
it would be to fuck him, get a lunch
money for a good month, work him
and mash him down, make him want
more and more, make him give all
him have — and then what would he say?
Wouldn't bother me. After all, that is how
that wicked man do me, and give me
this sickness. But I turn the corner
and gone. And you know, I see him

again one day, with his wife —
and I go to the wife and say, "You
should thank me, cause I coulda
kill you, and your husband just soh."
And she smile like she know,
and I walk my way. You see how
it hard to live right in this place?
Because I won't lie, is a nice looking
man, and what he said he wanted
to do with me, I wanted it, too,
my whole body saying yes, give me
some of that, and Savior, when him
say to me, "AIDS is nothing, make
we do it same way..." wrong as it is
to even feel like this, that was the cleanest
and most beautiful I ever feel since
I know, and I give thanks for that.

Untitled

Viet Lê

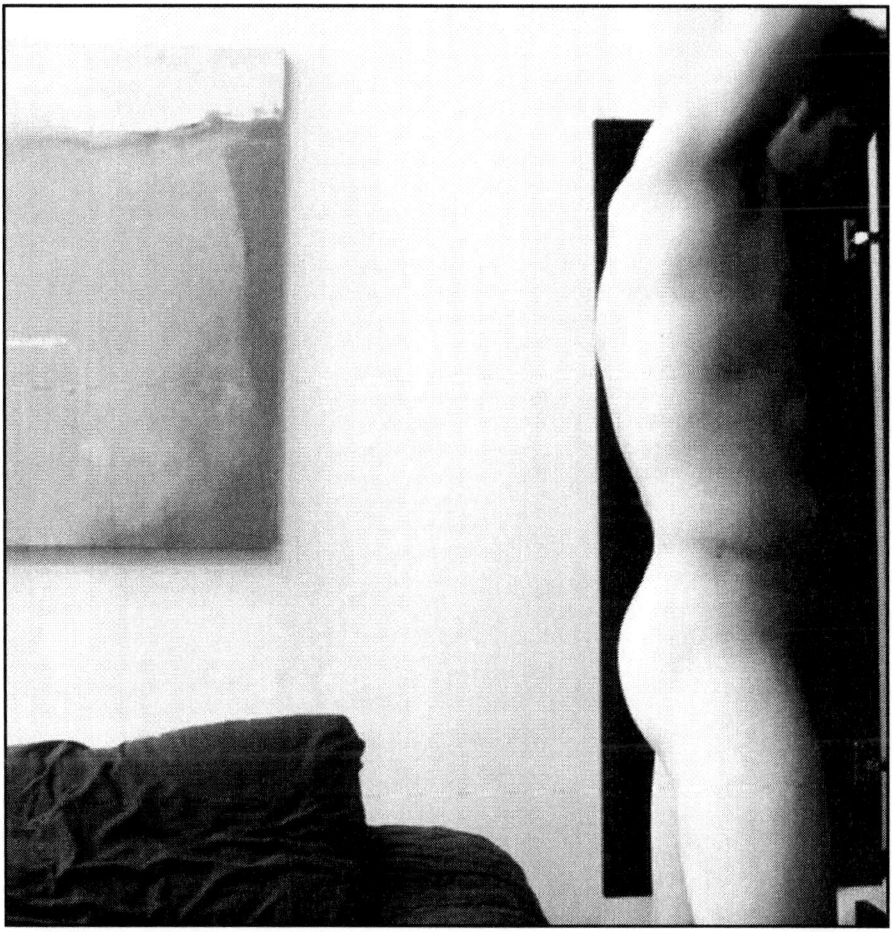

Atomic Weight Of the Soul
World AIDS Day 2008

Melissa Lippard

God's in particles they say.
Unproven
but if true,
too, then is he in ours?
The wait of possibilities
subcutaneous
and
of those who are well until
they
are not.

Our friends
Our daughters
Our sons
just grease smears on the lens.
Fractured light
off a chipped china sun
they bounce. Their light races
crashing back into sunlight until they are gone.
It didn't matter what they were,
but who.
In spite of what you may think,
like you,
they are made of the same dirt and blood and bone.

If souls have radiant weight,
in shining
soon, too, you to will be spun sand.
Ash and mud turned to translucent glass
in fire
that through you heats
until your light is no longer divisible by One
Soon, you will only be divisible by yourself.
A black hole where once you mattered.

The devil's in the details.
In the cells, too,
replicating
bastadarized dna,
Plucking out light by the handful,
weeding
until nothing is left but the
patch of dirt we started out as.
He can convince you
on a cellular
level to transform
into something unrecognizable,
microscopically unstoppable
cannibalistic —
until he is
digging 6 foot ditches
in your own soul.

Soon they may find answers,
either in a circuit of magnets and tubes
under Europe

Or in a microscoped spark of
ingenuity
that solves the cosmos in a Petri dish.
Will they then divine the weight of the soul,
glean the parts of its sum?
When they know what to add
or subtract
will they then reach for
the microscopic help of God,
or will they try to stop the devil's hand themselves?

If God
should be in our particles
he would then be there to straighten out viral RNA
His convexed power
flexing
light
back into perfection.
But maybe
He is too small to stop the onslaught.
Or maybe, in perfecting, His weight melts souls
like Shrinky Dinks
into concave glass
through which our
divergent light will scatter until none is left.

Recover/Discover

Richard Sawdon Smith

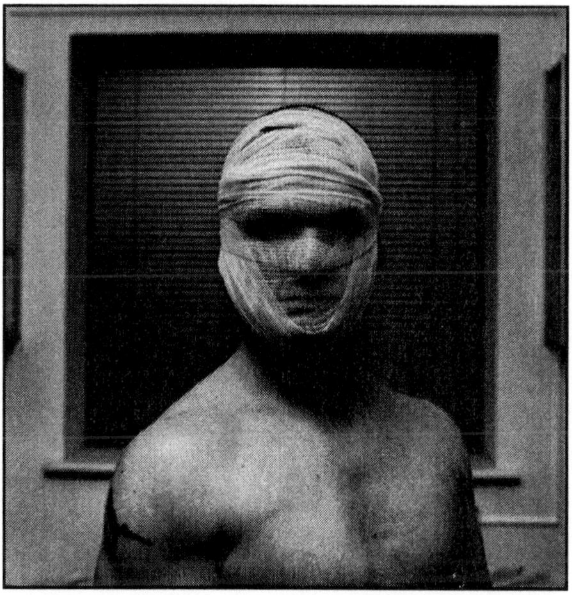

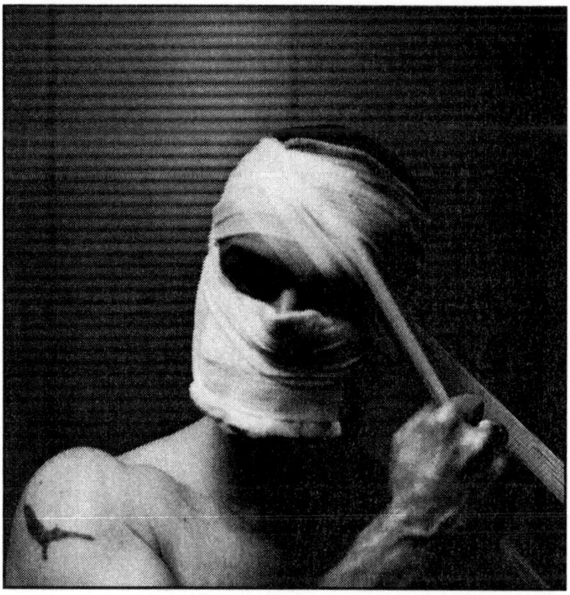

SECTION II
VIGIL

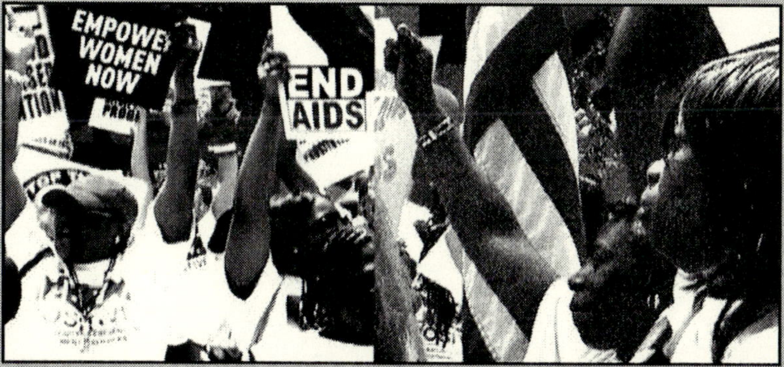

PROTEST | **Cyrille Phipps**

Vigil

for Floyd

Venus Thrash

Say artificial blessing
to late night bowl of cereal.

Hold vigil over computer keyboard
as if it's Floyd wasting on death's bed

in AIDS-induced coma
while Antonio and Todd

sing 'Happy Birthday'
over red velvet cake

Floyd will never get to eat.
In a cross-town apartment

blessed by Bearden,
Baldwin, Miles, Muddy,

Arthur tries to reconcile past sex
life with sunken face in mirror.

Hollow cheeks exhale thin air.
Fury rumbles the corners of his room.

Back home, sandalwood incense cascades
the apartment in sweet-smelling smoke.

Coltrane's *Isis and Osiris* intercourse
in the windless night.

Decide for tenth time
not to cut hair after all.

Roll another joint. Don't light it.
Try not to think about candles

burning all night for Floyd,
flesh taut on Arthur's bones—

light it anyway. Just two hits
and promise myself not to finish.

New Patients

for Hydeia Broadbent

Chanell Ruth

Since June 14, 1984, the day of her birth, Hydeia Broadbent has lived with HIV. At an early age she began speaking publicly about the disease while assisting her mother's activism, but eventually her voice overshadowed that of her own mother.

She gave
AIDS
a new face

brave
beautiful
Black
blistering
babies

Legendary

Emanuel Xavier

In memory of Pepper LaBeija

There are Gods amongst us in these ghettos
so black, so fierce,
so brown, so beautiful,
Their time on earth may be as oppressive as ignorance
limited to the demons flowing in their blood
but after safely passing over back to the clouds
the wind will still carry their auras and prophecies
their bones will still beat drums
for their children to dance
the phoenix will still rise from the flames of Paris
with hope in womb

There are Gods amongst us in these ghettos
so brown, so fierce,
so black, so beautiful,
If you spend too much time caught up in yourself
You just might miss Him that is goddess,
She that is god, they that are legends
Working the runway as if walking on water
Reaching the stage to that promised land
where 'peace' is not ridiculed
and the only war worth fighting for
is protecting your child from the terrorist acts
of a mainstream America
where 'reading' is an act of learning

not degrading words used to disguise fragility
and fractured dreams
where 'shade' is a shadow you walk in
to avoid the light
but who wants to stay out of the warmth of the sun?

If you waste your time trying to be a false prophet
robed in attitude and labels to obscure the insecurity
you may fail to recognize their divinity and miracles
parting the crowds, resurrecting from the floor,
scoring tens of commandments,
because trophies will not feed the hungry,
coat the homeless, hide the scars,
Grand Prizes will not bring Lazarus or LaBeija back from the dead
they will just sit in your closet,
fake idols gathering dust,
before the gold paint chips away
You cannot sell them for freedom
You cannot trade them in for love

There are Gods amongst us in these ghettos
so black, so fierce,
so black, so beautiful,
so brown, so fierce,
so brown, so beautiful,
Watch them carefully and say your prayers as they enter the ballroom
angel wing feathers decorating skin
recrafted over silicone and martyred colors
See the Gods dream, see the Gods give,
see the Gods live,
They exist in the spaces where white

is not the only hue that represents purity
They will not battle to your rhythms and beats
click, spin and dip simply for amusement
They will not teach those
who share their souls and names to hate
Their heartbeats are louder than the blaring speakers

You want realness . . . look at your hands
are they red from the revolution
or from the blood of your own sisters

There are Gods amongst us in these ghettos
so black, so brown, so fierce, so beautiful,
so bright
Look up towards the heavens and pray
then look at yourself in the mirror and say
'Stars are not only found out in the sky
but in ourselves'

Liberation

Shahari G. Moore

I remember when life was simple all laid out in black and white. No blurry grays clouded my mind, adding to my confusion. Right was right and wrong was wrong. I was either living on one side or the other. It was 1989 and house music in Chicago was giving Hip Hop a run for its money. On Friday nights I'd rock black Girbaud's, a leather Troop jacket, scrunch my high top under a Kangol, and wrap a bandana around my wrist. Breakin' was slowly stepping back in the Chi, but the rough and tumble spirit of Hip Hop remained. The teen parties on Friday night were filled with packs of pop lockers and head nodders, spinning to street anthems over rambunctious beats.

On Saturday nights I'd frequent Medusa's and celebrate the full glory of my high top fade. I'd wear polka dotted "Hammer" pants, striped shirts, and shiny shoes while twirling, pliéing, and sometimes splitting to House music. I loved both Hip Hop and House, but the latter art form seized my soul and made me feel like I had wings sprouting from my shoulders. On the dance floor I was free to be myself. There were few labels and judgment simply did not exist. Not even of men who spiraled around in each other's arms until they crashed to the floor.

The first time I saw him I fell in love. I'd never seen a man move like him. Watching him dance was like being baptized, the cool water running down my body after a frenzy of ring shouts and hallelujahs on Sunday morning. I made sure to keep my distance because he was unapologetically affectionate towards men and I simply wasn't ready. So I watched him dance as Pharris Thomas wrapped up his set. I watched him soul clap like thunder lived between his palms. He mouthed lyrics through full brown lips. "*You used to know how to love me right. You used to know how to love me ri-iight. You used to hold me...* "

I kept my eyes open and danced with caution, inching closer to him. Terry Hunter came on the turn tables and blended in, "*Just as long as I got you, I got enough...*" I danced near him, but not close enough to touch. Everyone knew that he was different and I wasn't quite ready for the world to know that I was different too. I tried to resist him, turning away from the whole of his beauty, but I succumbed and gave in to a truth that we both knew existed.

The raw honesty of his being encouraged me to let go of myself. Suddenly I broke free and didn't care. I felt the bass pounding inside my chest in sync with the beating of my heart. I let the feelings deep in my core express themselves through my limbs. I took in a deep breath and blew out my thoughts of the world and the world's thoughts of me. I spun around before him and bowed humbly in reverence from my gut. As I stood, our eyes met for the first time. I froze, wanting to stay in the moment, stealing time from past, present, and future. He soul clapped, acknowledged my performance, acknowledging me. He turned and walked away, carrying the bass and my heart. The lights came up signaling the party's end. I searched Medusa's for him, but I couldn't find him in the throng of Black bodies.

I woke up at 7:49 AM on Monday feeling, wanting, and needing to be seen by him again. My mother fixed grits and eggs for me with a little meat on the side. I picked at my grits, knowing that my hunger ran deeper than the food on my plate. I got up from the table, gave her a kiss, and made my way to the six. The number six bus reminded me of a snake, slithering and rattling along Stony Island. I'd never been one to trust snakes, but this one was faithful. It had gotten me to Hyde Park Career Academy on snowy days, hot days, and rainy days over and over again since I was a freshman. The six pulled up with one of those HIV posters on the side asking, "What if you were HIV Positive? Teach the World to Understand." I looked at the poster, rubbed the tension from my neck, climbed on, and paid my fare.

Hyde Park Career Academy was the best of both worlds, full of culture and opportunity, yet brimming with enough red and blue to get plenty of street cred from the Brutha's and the Folks on the south, west, and east sides of Chicago. As a senior, life felt different. I was painfully peeling back my own skin to see what lied beneath. And honestly a part of me was afraid to know who I really was. I sat through class and listened to Mrs. Murray pontificate on the sociology behind Spike Lee's, *Mo' Better Blues.* I could not stop thinking of my handsome prince and how I needed to be his Clarke and his Indigo.

After school I went to Dr. Wax on 53rd Street. I wanted to get the new Public Enemy and a Lil Louis mix. As I walked through the door there was something funny about the vibe. I made my way to the new releases and then I saw Aiesha near the Hip Hop section. Aiesha was a pretty, little chocolate girl with long skinny legs. She laughed a lot, loved to dance and seemed easy to talk to. She'd just broken up with Ray, a big burly dude on the football team with a gap between his teeth. Aiesha seemed cool, prom was coming up and I couldn't go by myself. As I walked toward her, I imagined how she'd look in a sassy satin dress with her hair stacked high in a fresh asymmetrical cut. I decided she'd look good. We'd look good together and my mother would be pleased.

As I got closer, she looked up and smiled. I smiled back as I felt the moistness gather under my arms. A girl like Aiesha would want to kiss and maybe more on prom night. My stomach tied itself into knots, but I had to ask her. Just as my hands began to shake, I heard it playing. *"You used to know how to love me right. You used to know how to..."*

I turned around and he gave me a subtle bow. He turned to the cashier and said, "I'll take it." The cashier stopped the tape, put it in the cover and bagged it up. "Alright Reese," the cashier gave him some 'dap' and Reese walked out of the door.

I waved bye to Aiesha as I heard the door chimes signaling my own exit. What was I doing? I wasn't quite sure, but I followed Reese down Lake Park to 48th street. He reached back and held the door open for me as he walked inside the building. As we waited for the elevator, an old lady sitting in the lobby cut her eyes at us and shook her head. We got on the elevator and got off on the seventh floor. I watched him walking down the hall. I loved the confidence in his walk. I wanted desperately for him to teach me to be me.

From the seventh floor I could see the crowns of the trees and feel the breeze blowing off Lake Michigan. I could see the people down below, but they couldn't see me. He challenged me to a game of Space Invaders and I sighed, relieved to hold onto the part of me who knew nothing about sex or being grown. Reese played mightily until he lost. As he passed me the joystick, I clutched his fist, touching him for the first time. I held onto his hand and stared into his face, noticing the flawless flow of each of his features into the other. Even the large mole on his cheek was worthy enough to be kissed. So I did as he stood up and walked over to the radio.

Reese played French Kiss for me and began to stir his pelvis in figure eights to the rhythm. He closed his eyes and eased his head back, lulled by the music. He reached for me and I met him in the dance, allowing sound to consume us. He caressed my face, looking deep into my eyes. The room became cool so he covered me with the warmth of his body. I turned toward the window, staring at the swaying trees. I searched for light between the spaces where the leaves and branches met. I watched the sun ease itself down, creating a blinding band of color across the horizon. I lost myself and found myself somewhere between the music and the sky.

A year passed and Hip Hop tattooed itself into society's skin. I'd gone back to Medusa's every chance I got during winter and summer break hoping to see Reese. College was cool, but sometimes I felt isolated as a gay male. I didn't put it out there; instead I just chose not to fit in. I never knew where Reese went after I graduated, but I figured no matter how far he'd gone he'd always have to come home. I missed his hands and I desperately needed to lay eyes on him once again. I went by Dr. Wax and asked the cashier if he'd seen him. He looked at me and sighed, "Sorry man, Reese died from pneumonia about six months ago. I heard he caught that shit." I got hot and felt as if I couldn't breathe. I tried to steady myself, feeling my knees give way. Then darkness came.

I woke up to the sound of Geraldo Rivera's voice and the touch of my mother's hand. "James, honey you've been passed out for almost four hours and the doctor is running some tests." The doctor came in shortly after that with my chart in hand. "Ms. Mills, could you please step into the hallway? I need to speak with James."

I reached for my mother's hand and whispered, "Stay." I watched the doctor's lips move, but all I could think about was the number six bus, slithering and rattling down Stony Island, the large mole on Reese's cheek, and the day I found and lost myself between the music and the sky. The doctor placed his hand on my mother's shoulder and she fell to the floor. That day I was diagnosed with H.I.V. at the spry age of eighteen.

If I could rewind my life I probably would choose not to. To edit my own awakening would be unauthentic. I will not apologize for being Black, gay, or male. I will not apologize for loving and receiving love the way that I saw fit. Everyday, life brings us one step closer to death. When I die, I will stand before God and confess that my greatest sin was not using a condom.

when my brothers fell

Raymond Berry

for Marlon, Joseph, Melvin, and Essex

after the quilt is tucked away promises
broken we will still be here wanting
answers for our deaths you passed on

your weapons now i use them without
questions chosen by need to continue what
you started stand where you once stood

bold, brave, ready

After the Care Conference

Julene Tripp Weaver

I. Skilled Nursing Home Discharge to Assisted Living

He lives in the zone
where he does not remember
being passed out on the floor
for two days in his condo.

No recollection of his friends finding him, or
the ambulance to the emergency room.
He was lucky, his friends had a key
prearranged out of concern.

He does not remember his week in intensive care
his transfer to this skilled nursing facility.

We remind him what is missing in his dementia,
You've lived at Bailey Boushay.
for three months now,
you have regular falls, incontinence.

His mind is full of large gaps.
A trial run with nurse supervision, proof
he does not take his meds as prescribed
he needs assisted living.

With much convincing he finally agrees.
This care team wants his health to return,

they come to these meetings, pay his bills.
know he cannot go home to fall again.

II. Ongoing Resistance once at Assisted Living

Thirty years of diplomacy, the Resident Coordinator
talks to families in distress, tries to gently impose
saving grace on minds etched with illness,
on those with a creeping virus that eats cells
taking memory with it. She talks slow,
asks the right questions direct:

Do you know how much these people care about you? Yes.
Do you know how sick you were? No.
Can you believe that these people who care about you will tell you the truth? Yes.
Will you take your doctor's advice? I will get a second opinion.
How long have you been with your doctor? A long time.
Do you trust your doctor? Yes.
Then will you consider making this decision after you get to talk with your doctor? Yes.

But he wants to go home to his condo
where the plumbing doesn't work.
He says, all it needs is a new sink, a new toilet.
He's lived there twenty years.

When the rent exemption stops
you will receive $58 each month,
not $600, not enough to cover a mortgage,
or your condo dues.

Never mind the needed repairs, basic utility bills and food.
He doesn't remember his business license lapsed,
that he does not have a phone anymore.
He thinks these problems will work out.
His outstanding credit debt totals thirty thousand.
He doesn't know how it got so high.

His friends and family live full lives;
one with a small child, another a whole parish,
a younger sister, a widow, afraid to put her foot down.
They found stacks of mail unattended over a year
a backlog of debt, lawsuits.

His condo is full of dusty books. His mind
a repository of information, insights to lives
he alone writes bibliographies on,
a whole encyclopedia of knowledge will slip away
if he doesn't receive daily care.

He doesn't know when his bowels move
or his urine flows, doesn't notice wetness
in his pants, but he talks of dead poets.

We repeat our mantra, his history of noncompliance.
We want him to maintain what he has gained,
help him to finish writing his book.

Behind his back we talk about guardianship,
futile against this inborn desire,
            independence at any cost.

Positive Voices of Dorm E

Rural Women's Health Project

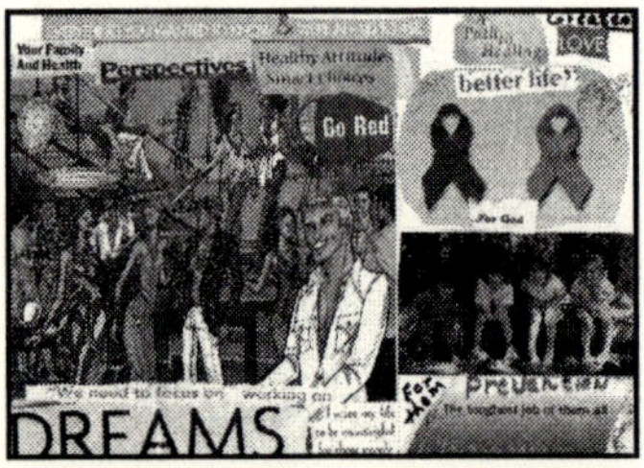

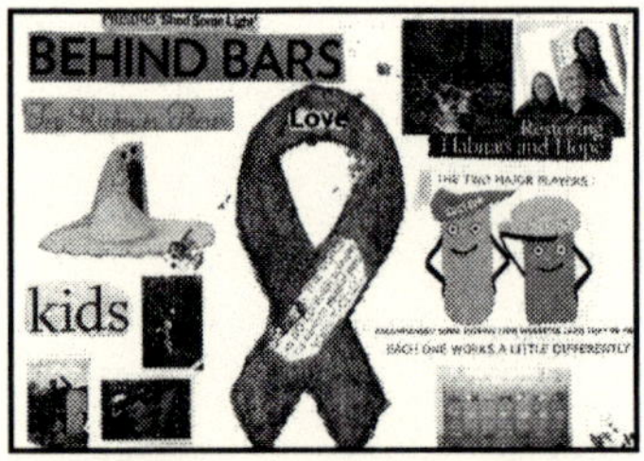

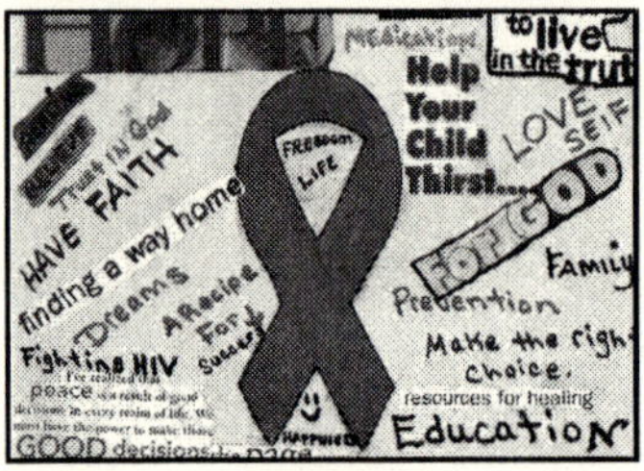

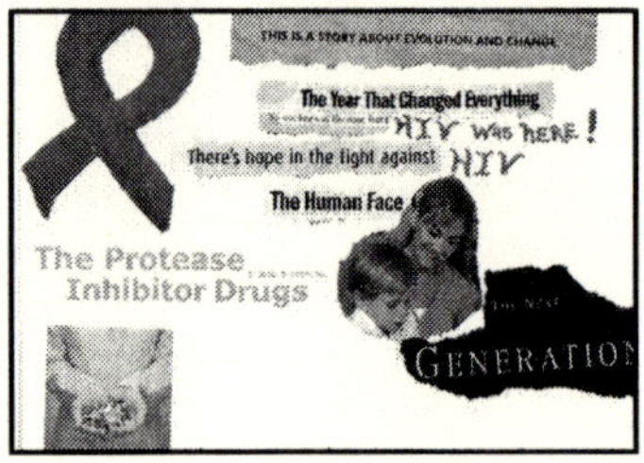

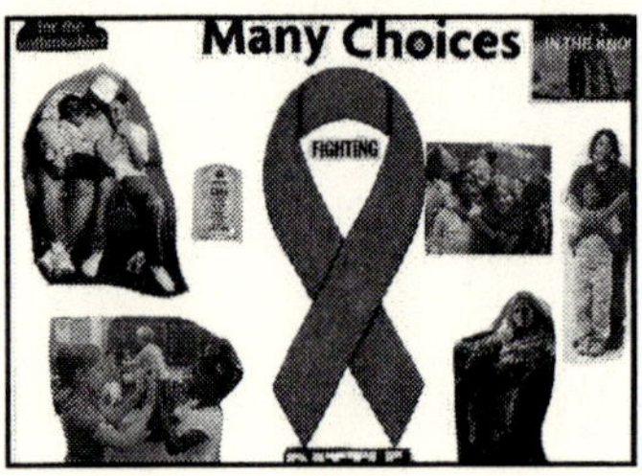

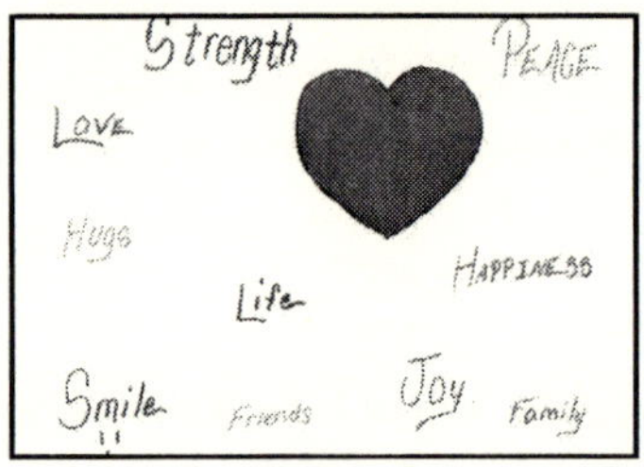

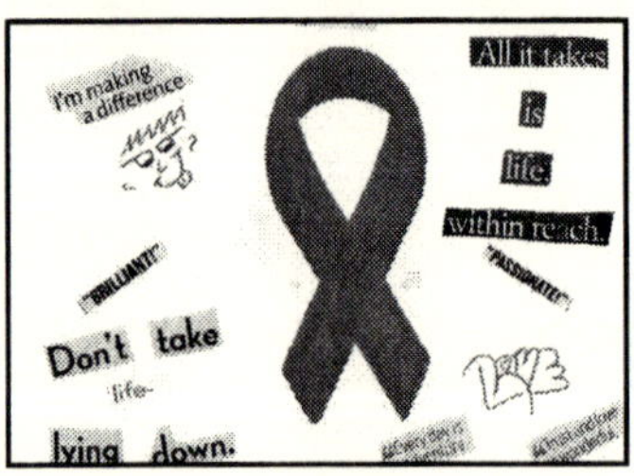

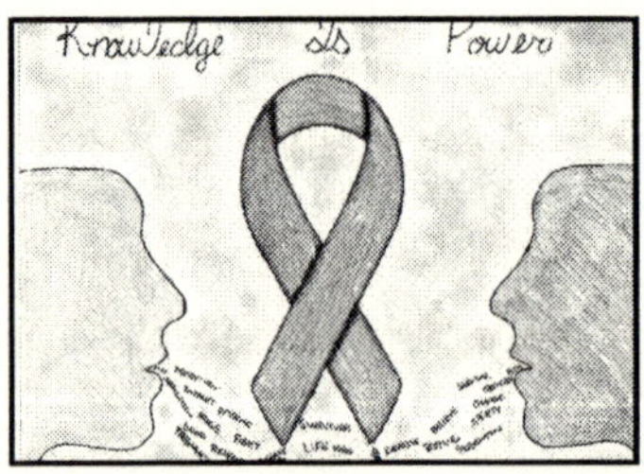

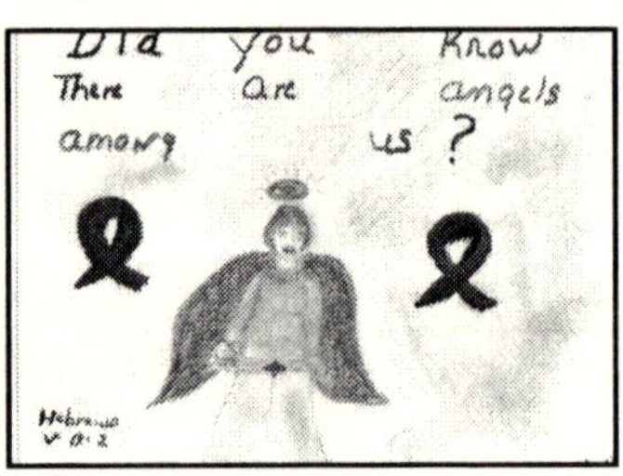

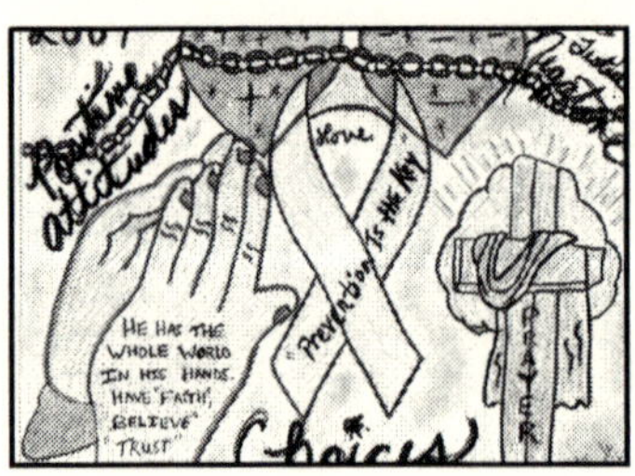

Quilt

Kwame Dawes

1

Powell

In the belly of this postcard city
a brown stench covers everything —
the ripeness of open sewers, the sweaty

narrow lanes, the horde of mumbling
people, the seediness of tourists' pleasures;
it is this dark earth and grime

that gave us the broken treasure
of a man, this sufferer counting time —
each hour — before the sickness dragged

him down. He taught us in the trick
of his smile the way to heal. This bag
of bones, this counterpoint to the tragic,

this was Powell, a brother whose passing
stung us like sea salt in the wind.

2

Margaret

Margaret, your mother gave you this yellow
name when the light was just right

and there was music slowly blowing
through the open louvres. While your bright

eyes drank her in, she fed you milk
and a future of loss, before she withered

away, before she grew slowly sick,
before she died. Margaret, did you remember

the name she gave you when her man
plowed into your infant womb the curse

in his blood, when he crammed
into your tender self, his anger and terror?

How can you now smile, little girl, how do you
carry this burden as if it's a wisp of dew?

3

Mango

Thanks for your appetite for ripe mangoes.
I washed them in caught rain water, wiping
them down, then cutting them into two
succulent cups. Thank you for the eating,

your mouth moving quickly, your body
savoring every sting of Bombay sweetsour;
thank you for gleefully sucking each seed
till it was white; thank you for the heat

on your gleaming head; the gurgling melody
of your pleasure; thank you that though
you became sick, yet you thanked me
for my gift to you. I pray that tomorrow

you will wake in mango heaven, feasting
on bushels of sweet, your renewed body shining.

4

Leaving

I would have wanted you to live longer,
but your healing came as forgiveness,
to doubt which would be to remember
the vomit you can't return to. The rest
of my days will be filled with me
trying not to forget, searching for a clue
of you in every ordinary thing — ackee trees,
a freshly picked June plum, the startling blue
of a three o'clock sky. I am still annoyed
with God for offering the lie of healing,
but he must know how to call his own
in his own peculiar way. All this leaving
is too much for me. You should have stayed,
my dear friend, that's all I know to say.

5

Quilt

Eventually, the expanding quilt grew too long
for the hall wall, and the stitching,

so hurriedly done, was no longer strong
enough to hold the fabric; the fading

initials fell limp, and folks were missing
their names. Five went last week, with no one

cutting strips of cloth, no one gathering
to hum prayers — they were just gone. Dying

has become ordinary and reminders are too much.
So we've moved the quilt to the store room,

folded it into a simple box. On the porch,
three simple candles burn, the gloom

of dusk broken by the vigil of flames;
in the trees' whisper you hear their names.

All Because New-Love Was HIV Positive

Randall Horton

slurred, the piercing drag of cold grinds
against beautiful wreckage — a blaring

out, new-love bleeds a tonic blue register,
smelling like just left bullets from the chamber,

she bemoans then moans metal daylight, it cuts
so badly, a fresh wound seethes, everything

china bright, the static color of confusion
gurgles in the brain why-o-why — officer

regarding he once liquidation of maleness:
into a woman's roseate sundress she slipped at nine,

but hatred that held the gun held hate,
now ain't life not grand to this passing lily, her petals

laying silently in falling snow is a flower.

what pashin flute told me

pashin flute her stripper name (of course)

avery r young

fo de ladies n gents who blow her

yo poet, i gotta man-man now. n dude know i like womens. dont mind at all, as long as i aint likin womens while him n me be together. but you know how dat go.

a couple thursdays back, i was pretzeled up with danni d. (my *stud* friend who be doin porn), n dude come bammin on de door. danni say *lets play 'we not here,'* but dude smell us. you know how dat go.

so to entertain danni, we play *we not here.* dude stop bammin. n when me n danni finish, i make danni leave out back door (just in case dude was playin *stop bammin on de door n just stand here, patiently, til dey come out).* half day later dude come bammin on de door agin, talkin bout, i got him fukked up. dude say him know i was wid some man-woman cause him had walked round, n watched me let 'it' out de back door from de alley.

now poet, i fukked up n let dick tracey in de house, but dat was to regain some peace — tween dude n danni, rent get paid. so i get all sweet n kiss him forehead real tender-like, n den i tell dude to cease wid all dat bullshit. but den, dude flip into *oprah winfrey* winfrey n wanna ax all type of questions. dude wanna know why i kiss *'it'* when i tell *'it' bye;* why i call *'it' 'boo bear'*; n why i smile when *'it'* walk down de stairs. n den dude goes into pointin out dat i dont do dat fo him. i go, *whatever dude, n what de fuk is an 'it'?*

n now i'm lookin at dude like him 14 yrs old n still in the 2nd grade, n dat look put dude on 10. so dude lay him hands upon my shoulders, n push me hard, n i hit de window, or de wall, or whateva.

n befo i cud put my mind on killin him to jee-sus, him say some shit like *what other nigga gonna want yo corroded nutbox?*

you want it, i say befo erything turn into pitch black-ed-ness. n when i regain my natural self, dude pleadin with poe-poe to let him go grab somethin i need really bad befo dey take me to de station. i focus n see dude left eye swole shut n him shirt bleevin. *oooo weee! what did i do* is what i wanna say, but *dude put him hands on me first,* all dat come out. but i might as well be a mime to dem muddafukkas cause all dey hear is dude swole shut left eye n bleevin shirt.

den poet, dat dude come back outta my house wid my bottle of meds tween him thumb n pointy finger, n say, here. *take dis. dat bitch likes to spread it like mayo.*

erybody outside gettin a good heapin helpin of neo-nigga theatre n i cant believe himll put my bidness all out on karlov like dat. *dude put him hands on me first,* i say one mo time fo de def dumb n blind officer who keep pushin my head into de squad car.

n befo i know it, de bark in me reaches up, n bites down.

The News in Spring

Remica L. Bingham

—after Marilyn Nelson and Elizabeth Alexander

Words battle the car stereo, rushing air, evening traffic—
what good is the approaching summer, what good the trip
east and uncle's open arms at Gate 40, Terminal B,
what good the shared straw in a Watermelon Freeze
passed between rocking chairs at Friendly's, what good
his homeruns on Red Bank Field two blocks
from Count Basie Theater, what good the live jazz
Friday evenings on the water, what good the crisp
twenty dollar bill pressed into my palm for
whatever, those books you like, what good the stories
about his escapades, his four women at my parents'
wedding, what good the mystery, the rumored
clairvoyance, birth with a veil and two teeth,
what good his premonitions when—*Your uncle*
Ralph
AIDS

Names (Those Who Lived and Died with AIDS)

Nina Bennett

At first it is easy to remember the names of those who died. I speak confidently at the candle lighting—Stephen.

One year three men died in a row. First Doug. His sister didn't want his ashes so we defiantly scattered them at his favorite cruising spot. Then Tommy, who dragged his portable oxygen tank outside while he smoked. Finally John. I wailed at his funeral as his majestic tenor sang Ave Maria on a tape from his sister's wedding.

Frank's father pissed me off when he preferred drug overdose be listed as his son's cause of death.

Then there was the year people fidgeted when the names kept coming. In a sing-song chant I called them out, like naming the plagues at Passover. Marvin. Jack. Moe. Butch. Locusts. Frogs. Anna. Elaine. Jimmy. Darkness. Hail. Lloyd. Nancy. Disease. That was the last candle lighting I attended.

Jeff wanted to use me as a model and cut my waist long hair in a shag. Two years after he died I cried at the swish of scissors and closed my eyes as the long strands floated to the ground.

Eventually I couldn't recall all the names. I sat on the floor with the bottom file drawer pulled open, the one without a typed label; manila folders precisely lined up like soldiers on the parade ground. Our secretary was afraid to touch them.

Chucha's Last Christmas

Tony Medina

No more vacant lot eyes staring
    Blankly into your future

You used to dream of being a dancer
    Of letting your heart move

Along your *nalgas*
    Along the island of your pulse

O what rhythms wrestled through
    Veins of coke & heroin

& frustrated despair
    Of being a Black Puerto Rican

Woman *una negra* unsatisfied
    In her captive world

How you wanted to *merengue* the
    Shit out of those motherfuckers

& let 'em know what it
    Be's like

Chucha, there are no more
    Long nights in welfare hotels

No more selling dreams
  At the OTB or

Lifetimes & lifetimes
  Spent in a bottle

Dangling between
  A needle & a vein

No more lives &
  Times & dreams

& pains rolled up in
  Bambu paper

You used to walk
  Those winter nights

Alone stone cold
  In your salsa blues

& your wetness turning to
  Icicles in your

Drawers dreaming of
  Eating *pasteles*

In your grandma's
  House

Those days are
  Over now, Chucha

Who was to know
  That you would

Hug the third
  Rail

& who could
  Blame you?

Gunpowder Lives

Venus Thrash

for Tim and Kenneth and their mothers

Ever since that night in November
when my next-door neighbor stopped
in front of the stoop and unfolded
the Post to her son's smiling face,
I have been obsessed with the Obits page.

Here, she says, handing me the paper,
pointing to a picture of her son, Kenneth,
who had been shot down *like a damn dog*
two years ago that day. No words can soothe
in the presence of her dead son.

Her round shoulders tremble and bounce.
Her eyes flood over.
Nadine and Mary offer her a shoulder,
a well-smoked blunt, a double shot
of Christian Brothers brandy.

She takes a hit, declines the booze,
drags her dead son's damp face
up a desolate flight of stairs.
Nadine and Mary beg her not to go up
to that *sad, empty-ass apartment.*

But she ascends and disappears behind
a wall of cinderblocks. Nadine whispers,
It's time to let him go a little. Yeah, Mary says,
blowing smoke past my eyes, long as she keep
his room just like he left it, she gonna always

be breaking down over him. I say nothing
of my own grief for my dead friend, Tim,
his last photo lying on the backseat of my car,
his sunken eyes asking questions no one
can answer. I toss heartbreak aside

like the funeral program that has been riding
around with me since he died, past Ron's Unisex
Barbershop where I got my first Philly high-top fade
and Tim got his coif retouched and curled, past
Carnegie Library where we both cruised the men.

Between relic rides through the streets
of Washington, a hit on the blunt,
and a shot of brandy, snapshot images
of Tim and Kenneth strobe through my mind
like contractions three minutes apart.

Born on nights celebrated in violence,
firecrackers in their mothers' wombs,
gunpowder lives lasting 33 and 18 years
until they lit up the sky like making risky
love and a callous gunshot in the night.

I read the Obits as front-page news,
scan the photos of well-trimmed goatees
on boyish faces, examine the headstone years
etched in ink, sum of their lives as a lack
of longevity enshrouded in the morning edition.

Title Card

Cyrille Phipps

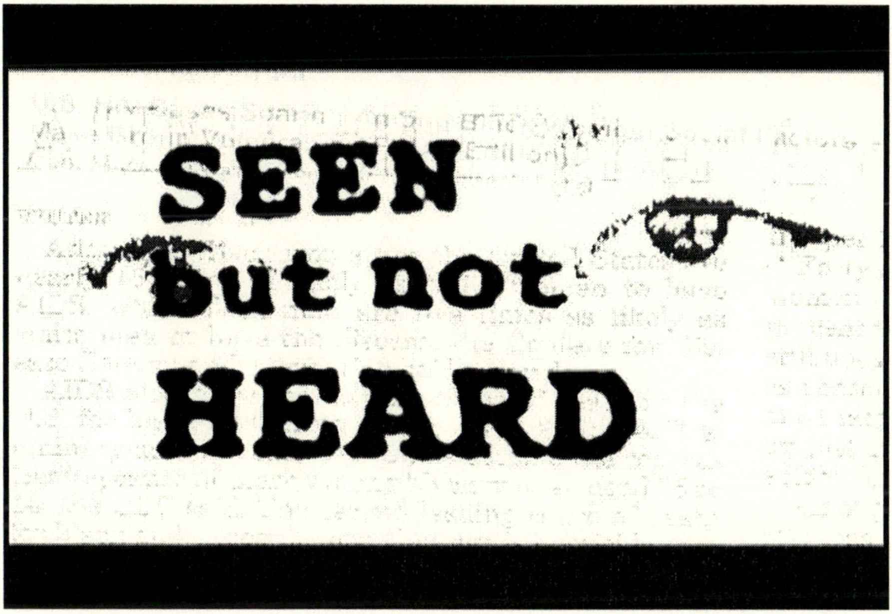

Guillermo's Lion

John Kotula

One of the first things I did when I arrived in Sonaguera, Honduras as a Peace Corps volunteer was to help out with the vaccination campaign. I went around to the villages with a team from the health center. We set up mainly in schools. In the village of Cuyulapa we had a busy morning, but by afternoon things had slowed down. I took a break to look around the school, introduce myself to the teachers and try out my Spanish on the kids. The school had a large assembly room and looking through the windows I saw some pretty good murals painted on the walls; portraits of historical figures, the national flower and national tree, the Honduran flag and the official seal, probably all copied from a civics text book.

I asked the director who had done them and she said a man named Guillermo from Arenas, the next village over. I said I'd like to meet him and the director grabbed a passing kid and sent him off on a bike to find Guillermo. I learned later it was about a five mile bike ride to his house. I don't think the kid ever made it back to school that day and Guillermo had not shown up by the time I headed back to Sonaguera. I had his name and knew his village so I figured I could look him up after the vaccination campaign. However, when I got to the Health Center the next morning he was waiting for me, having ridden his bike forty minutes from Arena. He was a small, thin, handsome man, wearing a green long sleeved shirt, way too big for him, buttoned up to the throat. We went across the street for a soda and what passes for a conversation given my level of Spanish.

I managed to tell him that I was an artist and wanted to meet artists in the area. I hoped in the future we could work together to present information about health issues such as HIV/AIDS. He was quiet and deferential, but clearly interested in what I was saying. He told me that his usual work was cutting oranges, but that whenever he had the chance he painted.

He had some drawings with him that he unrolled one at a time to show me. There was a lion lying on the bank of a river, a dove spreading its wings above a bible, an unfinished, imaginary city of domes, arches and towers. My two favourites were portraits; one of a man in profile wearing a cowboy hat and the other a delicately drawn frontal view of a young man with his collar buttoned up just like Guillermo's. They weren't good drawings in any technical sense, but like the paintings in the school, they were sweet and endearing and I liked them a lot.

We agreed to meet every couple of weeks to look at each other's drawings and to talk. He showed up two weeks later. I showed him my sketchbook and took a photo of him that I later used as a source to do a portrait. He didn't make our third meeting, but I wasn't worried because I figured he'd be easy enough to find if I could develop the opportunity to work together.

About three weeks later, my wife Deb and I were walking toward the Health Center in the early evening. It had cooled a bit and the sun was setting. A man came up behind us, touched my arm and said, "Excuse me. The boy in the car wants to talk to you."

He pointed to a pick up parked a few yards behind us. Guillermo was sitting in the passenger seat. I knew it was him right away, but I was disoriented because the change in his appearance was so dramatic. My first reaction was that he looked much younger, like he must have looked as a boy. Then I realized that he was very sick and had lost so much weight it was as if he had shrunk to a smaller version of himself. It was also disorienting to shake hands with him because his touch felt so much hotter than you expect a human touch to feel.

"Guillermo," I said. "You're sick."

"Yes," he said. "My problem is AIDS."

He told me that he had been to a doctor in Tacoa. I couldn't understand what the doctor had said or what the plan was. I think I asked if he was going to the hospital and he said, "Not yet." He was having trouble holding his head up and talking. I tried talking to the other men, his older brother, Eulalio, and his neighbor, Jose, about the hospital and about medicine and I think I kept getting "not yet" as an answer.

Finally, I made arrangements to visit him at his home on Monday. They told me to stop at Jose´s house, across from the Catholic Church and he'd show me the way.

Three days later, I found the neighbor´s house easily. While I was waiting for him to rouse a teenage son to show me the way to Guillermo's, I noticed a large painting on the kitchen wall. It showed an elegant and peaceful lion walking through a lush jungle. I knew right away it was Guillermo's. It had the same sweet and endearing qualities as his other pictures, but this was also a good painting, large, vivid, well rendered and personal. I was willing to bet that it wasn't a generic lion, but was in some way meaningful to Guillermo. It was my hope to get the chance to ask him about it.

I walked a half mile or so up the road with the neighbor´s son, sharing the road with cows, horses, pigs and bicycles, over a skinny log spanning a small stream, the only way across with dry feet if you were walking. I think I must have been the first gringo to pass through Arena in awhile. My presence was drawing more attention than it does in Sonaguera.

We walked through orange groves for ten minutes and then turned up a path leading into a packed dirt yard where a family was cooking and washing in front of a small cinder block house. I talked for awhile with a man who turned out to be Guillermo's younger brother visiting with his family from Tacoa. He told me Guillermo was worse, that he couldn't talk, that he was confused, but that he wanted to see me. We walked up a pretty path, further back into the orange grove, to another small house.

Guillermo lived here with his mother and two of her grandchildren, the teenage son and daughter of a sister of Guillermo's who had died. It was clear that the life of the family took place in the yard where there is a wood burning mud stove, a table, a pila (all purpose sink), and shade. The house was just for sleeping. It had two rooms with two beds in each room. In the back room the diminutive Guillermo was sleeping. I knew he was 31, but he looked 12. Once again my main reaction was one of disorientation. How could it be that just a month ago he road his bike forty minutes each way to visit me in Sonaguera?

He woke up, sat up, gestured to his mouth, his right arm, his right leg. His brother told me his right side was sleeping. I held his hand and it was still feverish. I gave him the photograph and the portrait I had drawn from it. His mother came in to look at them, too. I thought, *she has lost one child I know of, the dead daughter, now her son is dying.*

She was probably younger than I am. I said to the brother I'd just met that Guillermo had to go to the hospital. He said I had to wait and talk to his older brother. Just a couple of minutes later, Eulalio came in. He had a form, a paper from the Health Center in Tocoa. It said that Guillermo had a positive HIV test two years ago. It was a referral to Hospital Atlantida in LaCeiba, three or four hours away by bus, the only place where retro-viral treatment was available.

The family was gentle and loving. They lived in the middle of a beautiful orange grove. They had no money, no car. Their brother weighed 90 pounds. His right side was sleeping. He needed to go to the hospital. He was too weak to change buses twice, wait an hour in between in the sun on the highway; besides there was no money. Three teenage nephews were on the peripheral listening to the discussion about their dying uncle.

I asked about the neighbor and his truck. There was no money for gas. I offered to pay for the gas. Eulalio and I went to talk to the neighbor. It was possible. He had health problems too: pains in his stomach and back. It was a long drive, but for 800 lempira it was possible. We made the deal. They would stop at my house at 5:30 the next morning on their way to the hospital with Guillermo.

When Eulalio and I got back to their house, Guillermo was sitting up in the yard. His younger brother was feeding him small bites of Cup-O-Noodles. I went home with a sack of oranges and two small paintings of Guillermo's, a portrait of Francisco Morazan, a Honduran hero who almost united Central America in the 1830s and another of Francisco Ferrera, independent Honduras´ first elected president.

Paying 800 lempira for gas was charity, not development. It was not what the Peace Corps is about. It was not sustainable. I couldn't personally fund the transportation of every AIDS patient in Honduras. At the time, it felt like the best fifty dollars I ever spent.

It may be that since the night Guillermo's brother touched my arm in the street, the family was waiting for me to help. There is the possibility that they saw being acquainted with the gringo as their best resource. When I asked if they were going to the hospital and they said, "Not yet," that may have meant, "Not until you help us." They never asked, but should I have figured out sooner what was needed from me?

The next time I saw Guillermo he was in the AIDS unit at Hospital Atlantida in LaCeiba. In a room full of men, maybe fifteen of them, who looked like they were dying, he looked the closest to death. Deb and I had introduced ourselves to Dr. Flores, the director of the AIDS treatment program. He was friendly and generous with his time. He talked to us in his office for a half hour answering all our questions. We also saw him be kind and attentive to patients and family, including Guillermo's brother.

I felt, immediately that, given the limitations of the system, Guillermo was in good hands. Dr. Flores accompanied us and Eulalio up to the ward to see Guillermo. His hospital johnny had ridden up exposing his stick legs and underwear. His big brother tugged it back down covering him better. His head was bandaged. There was blood on his sheets and on the floor. He had fallen out of bed. Dr. Flores made arrangements for Eulalio to have a pass to the ward so he could stay with Guillermo and take care of him. There was not enough staff to watch him, feed him, help him go to the bathroom. Dr. Flores roused Guillermo. He may or may not have recognized me. He fell back asleep immediately. Later, he looked dead. I couldn't tell if he was breathing or not. Eulalio must have been thinking the same thing. I saw him lay his hand on his brother's chest to reassure himself.

Dr. Flores said the paralysis and cognitive dysfunction are from toxoplasmosis. It was in his brain. If they could get it under control, he would be a good candidate for retro-viral therapy. The retro-viral treatment was funded, but more immediately he needed a CAT scan to see how much brain damage there had been. There were no funds for this. It cost 3,000 lempira. Monday the social worker would start looking for the money. If we could give something it would be a big help. Dr. Flores was very direct for a Honduran. Later, Deb and I came back with 1,000 lempira from our account in the states.

That night in our hotel room, as I was falling asleep, I asked Deb what if the CAT scan showed so much brain damage that they decided he was not a good candidate for retro-viral treatment? What if my involvement helped keep him alive, but the paralysis was permanent and he couldn't cut oranges or paint? What if his mother and brother had to care for him as an invalid?

Guillermo died on June 29 at 10:00 in the morning. He got well enough to leave the hospital and travel home, but quickly became very ill again. He died six days later. Eulalio sent word to us that he had died and the hour of his death. It was understood that he would be buried 24 hours later.

When Deb and I arrived at the Evangelical church in Arena, only his mother, sister-in-law, and niece were there. They had been with him all night. The inside of the church was dim and cool compared to the glare of the street. The casket seemed impossibly narrow. It was wood, painted gray and white. There was a rough handrail screwed to the side for lifting it. About a quarter of the top was hinged and opened to reveal a Plexiglass viewing plate. There was no pretense that the casket held anything other than a corpse. A white towel hooded Guillermo's skull like head. There was cotton in his mouth and nose. His eyes and lips were slightly opened. I looked at him for a while and remembered other deaths, my mother, Deb´s dad, Gerry MarAurelle, Francis Giambroni. There was a smell. Clearly, it was time to get him into the ground. Right at 10:00 the church filled up, probably 50 people arrived within 10 minutes, including Eulalio.

He talked with us awhile. It came up that he had been looking for a camera. I had put mine in my pocket that morning, thinking that if there was time, I would take pictures of the painting of the lion. I agreed to take pictures of the funeral including ones of Guillermo's corpse.

I helped carry the casket from the church to the back of a pick-up. It was very light. There were two other pick-ups and the fifty or so people all piled in. The funeral procession was three pick-ups and a group of maybe fifteen people on bikes following behind.

The cemetery was just past the family's house, down a dirt path, through an orange grove. Guillermo's grave had been dug in the shade of a large tree, right next to where his father was buried. Four men carried the casket from the truck to the grave and put it down on the ground. Eulalio opened the lid so people could look through the Plexiglass again. He signaled me to take pictures. In these photos, Guillermo was visible but there were also reflections of the trees and sky above him. In Spanish the word for sky and heaven is the same: cielo.

The minister arrived and stood on the mound of dirt that had come out of the grave. He said that there is no need to pray for Guillermo because he has gone to his real life, his eternal life. He is with Jesus in glory and will be forever. The minister had a kind voice. While he was speaking his young son was standing just below him on the mound of dirt, tossing pebbles toward the grave.

A nephew jumped down into the grave and with a coffee can bailed out water that had seeped in. The men worked out the logistics of the ropes and lowered the casket into the grave. It took some doing to get the ropes free and pull them back out. The children all came up to the edge of the grave and threw in handfuls of dirt from the pile. Then the men shovelled. There were three shovels and they relieved each other silently. It probably took twenty minutes to fill the grave.

Eulalio had arranged for the pick-up that carried the casket to take us back to Sonaguera. He rode along with us.

That night as we were falling asleep in our bed, I asked Deb if, in the end, it would have been better if Guillermo had never gone to the hospital, if he had just stayed home with his family and died a month earlier.

Later, I asked Eulalio if people knew his brother had died of AIDS. He said no. I asked him if the family knew. He said no. I knew that people knew, because when they learned that I knew Guillermo they told me he died of AIDS. I knew the family was aware because I had been part of conversations about his illness with everyone in the family present. I took Eulalio's answer to mean it was something we don't talk about. It was not acknowledged.

After Guillermo died I sought out his artwork and photographed it. There was a surprising amount. The Catholic Church in Sonaguera had two beautiful easel paintings. There was a large mural in an Evangelical Church in Barrio Veintecinco. Deb came across another painting of a lion in the house of a midwife she was interviewing. I heard of several others as far away as LaCeiba. Having these images was important to me.

Deb and I went back to see Dr. Flores, the director of the AIDS treatment program where Guillermo was hospitalized. I had printed out a photo of Guillermo's Lion for him. We waited to see him in the pharmacy at the hospital where he was giving out prescriptions. He was working in an office separated from the waiting room by a curtain. He noticed us and nodded, but finished with his patient. I said to Deb, half joking, "He thinks we came to ask for our money back."

He did in fact explain to us that it had been too late to use the donation to get a CAT scan for Guillermo. He said we could either have the 1,000 lempira back or he would keep it and use it to help another patient. We said to keep it and I gave him the photo. He started crying quite hard. None of us could talk for a while. He must see so much death. I respect him greatly for doing the work he does and somehow managing to stay emotionally alive.

It seems to me, that as an artist, Guillermo had the ideal relationship to his community. He made it a more beautiful place, decorating homes, schools and churches. He helped people pay attention to things they might not otherwise have noticed. He was a man that the community couldn't afford to lose so young. It stuck with me that if my work in Honduras could in any small way prevent premature deaths it would be time well spent.

I never got to talk to him about his lion.

Doctor, One Day I Found a Cure

Michelle Mashon

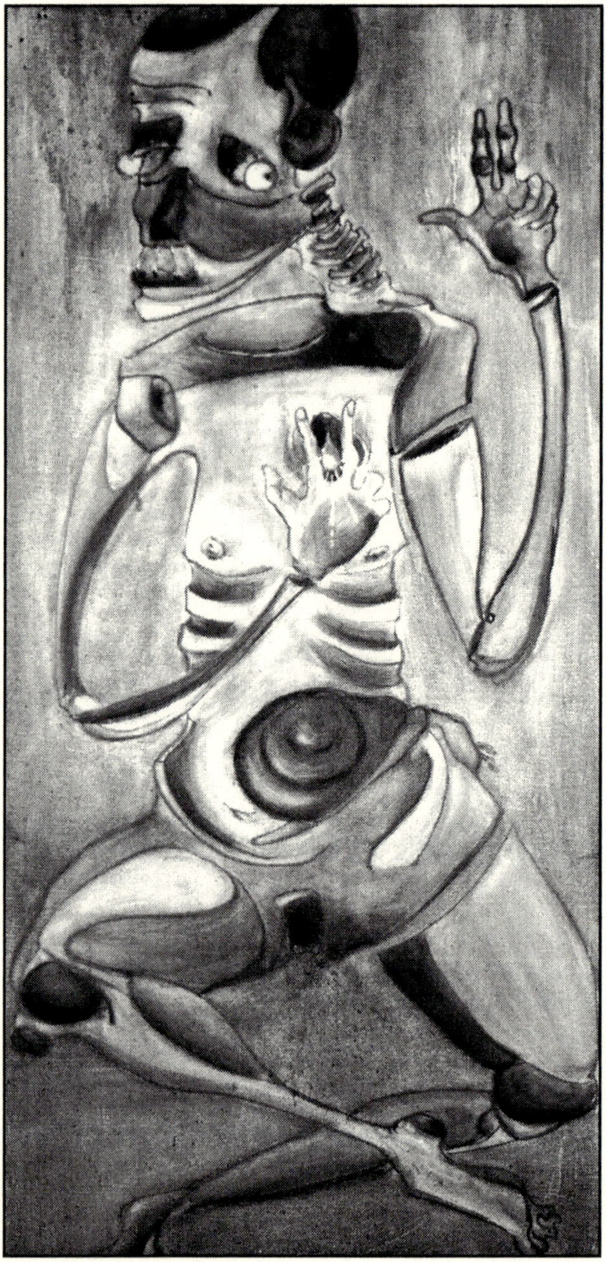

New York Citied

Ellen Hagan

for Greg

At Cedar Tavern on University,
we down pints of Hoegarten
which I've never tasted before,
but that isn't saying much. I am
new. Greg squeezes lemons inside,
lights eleven cigarettes. Marlboro
and sits way back in the church
pews for seats, we are religion.
Grad school year one, and we are
a kind of crew. Holy. His acne,
scarred skin, pockmarks, I am 23 and
it's New York City. And I am drunk
We are a wash. I have a crush on two boys
in our class. They are writers too. Greg is in
love with them both. We discuss their merits
over gin and tonics and piles and piles
of french fries. The twin towers have just
fallen. I always feel broken. Greg is
always next to me. He is a kind of healing
I have never known.

It's December and cold at the bar
below Three of Cups before Greg

will say, over pitchers and shots of Maker's,
after the weird holiday party, and we drive
in an unfamiliar car around the East Village
where I don't know it, but I'll live in two years
when he'll tell us, drunk and laughing that he hopes
the pneumonia doesn't come back. "I couldn't take it
then. Too many hospital trips, trauma, time in gowns,
and you know me, under sheets, covered up, and you
know me." Always a cough raging that winter. Below
chest. Disappearing. "God, fuck. Feel like
I've had this thing for years," and more laughing. His hack,
routine. Another drink. Cigarette. His hand on my knee.
That night etched for me. Kisses, night.

Then it changes. Because it always ends up
doing that. Because he did get pneumonia again.
What fails the body. Corrupts. What gives. Immunity
down. The system. Blown. How it flips, and then turns
itself all inside. What gives. What gives. What plants
and then grows. Is internalized. Brutal.

The last story we read in class,
was his carnival story. His first kiss
with a boy. He read without crying.
Straight through. His grin. Seduction.
The boys I loved loved him too. Course, he
wore leather jackets and slim jeans, his hair
slicked just right. Could write. My God
he could write.

At the memorial that's all I could say. I wanted
to say more. There was always more. Say how we
talked from 6th Avenue all across town. How he saved me,
kept my country-ass in his city. 20 years, his city,
what was home. What he did, how he did it.
They knew. I know they knew. We all knew too.

After the Last Breath

Alice Myerson

We gave a toothbrush to his cousin
to smooth his downy scalp.
His sister wrapped
a doo-rag round his head,
and wove three locks of hair
into a soft translucent braid.
The nurse removed the lines
and washed his lifeless limbs
with lanolin.
His mother
closed his eyes.
"Does your chest hurt?"
we asked with some concern
"Mi corazon se muerte,"
she said,
her mouth still twisted from the stroke.
The season lost its order on that day,
and spring
stabbed winter with
a wrinkled, autumn leaf.
We searched for words of solace
to explain the emptiness of grief.
"God only gives you a burden
you can bear."
"He's in a better place."
"With God,
you know,
he's suffering

no more."
"The virus too
is dead,
let it be said."
Before his time,
and yet it was his time.
So,
let us imagine
him,
that frail, defiant boy,
sliding down a rocky stream,
somewhere between two great and giant hills,
on the other side of the earth,
in California,
his doo-rag flapping in the wind.
The trees would have bowed to him
with applause from the birds
A South Bronx boy on a white-water raft.
His eyes would have been
round
and brown.
His hoodie
would have fallen off his shoulders
and his thin hands
would have reached out
to grab
the sun.
It must have been marvelous
to hear his wry street smile
fill the woods
with boyish laughter.

The Unanswered Questions

Beatrice M. Hogg

Ever since I was thirteen years old, my cousin Richard "Dickie" Person had been my role model. He was stylish, sophisticated, and worldly, traits I hoped one day to acquire.

I met Dickie at my mother's funeral in 1970 and saw him again at my father's funeral in 1975. After that, I visited him regularly in Baltimore, Washington, D.C. and Harrisburg. He was the first person I knew who had a grand piano, sang Italian opera, collected artwork and traveled around the world. He showed me that there was more to life than the small coal mining community where I grew up. Every visit with him was a learning experience.

Dickie's birthday was January 3, the day before mine. He understood me better than any of my other relatives. Maybe that was due to our Capricorn connection. He was the only one who encouraged me to follow my dreams. Only Dickie understood why I moved from Pennsylvania to California when I was thirty-one. When I ran out of money during my first month in San Francisco, Dickie loaned me $500. With his support, I was able to make it until I got a paycheck from my new job.

Even though we were 3,000 miles apart, we kept in touch by telephone. In 1992, I went to visit him in Harrisburg. He took me out to dinner. It was the last dinner we ever shared. Later that evening, Dickie and I went for a ride in his Pontiac Fiero sports car. He took me to his secret apartment in another part of town, miles away from the home he shared with his disabled mother. Since the bedroom was the only room that was furnished, I knew he kept the apartment so he would have a place to bring men.

During my early twenties, I realized that Dickie was gay. Even though I had grown up in a small town, I wasn't shocked by this discovery. It explained the young, good-looking men that were always around him whenever I came to visit. Maybe it also explained his good taste in decorating and clothes. But all that I cared about was that he was happy and healthy.

I kept him informed about my life in California. I would send him copies of my published articles. In March 1994, I called his office and found out that he was on a leave of absence. When I called him at home, he would not tell me the nature of his illness, only that he was having "good days and bad days."

Around 10 PM on July 13, 1994, I got a call from our cousin Bonita. Years ago, she and Dickie had purchased a house together in Baltimore. That house had been the site of many of my happy memories of Dickie. Bonita and Dickie had always been very close. I wondered why she was calling me so late, as it was 1 AM in Maryland.

"Marvella," she said, "I called to tell you about Dickie."

Bonita sounded different, more distant than usual. I wondered what was wrong. "What about Dickie?"

"Well, you know that he has been sick, right?"

I was afraid of what she was going to say. I tried to keep my voice from shaking. "Yeah, I talked to him in March. He said that he was sick, but he wouldn't say what was wrong."

There was silence on the other line. Why couldn't Bonita tell me what was wrong?

"Dickie has AIDS, Marvella. He is dying. If you want to see him alive, you should go back to Pennsylvania soon. He doesn't have long to live."

The room seemed to disappear. "Okay," I heard myself saying. "I have to go home for my class reunion next month. I'll go to visit him then. Thanks for letting me know."

I blindly placed my phone back in its cradle. I took off my glasses and rubbed my eyes to wipe away the tears. "Not Dickie," I said to myself. Why did it have to be Dickie? I had heard about AIDS, I had read about AIDS, but I had never in a million years thought that it would ever affect my life.

I was stunned. I was paralyzed. The world became blank and futureless. I could not imagine a future without the smiling, positive presence of my dear Cousin Dickie. What would I do without him? How did this happen? Dickie was a registered nurse; he had a master's degree in nursing administration. How could he have been so stupid, so careless?

My heart was breaking. Both of my parents had died, but they both had been in their seventies and ill for a long time. Dickie was only fifty-three. He should have been entering the best years of his life. I started to cry even more, mourning the one remaining love of my life.

The next day, I called my friend Reuben. He was gay, and his brother was HIV positive. I knew Reuben would understand what I was going through. He gave me the support and comfort I needed to go on. I called my best friend Mary and told her the news. She had met Dickie once in Harrisburg. He had gotten tickets for us back in 1986 when the Grateful Dead had played in Hershey. She remembered his warmth and friendliness. Like Reuben, she didn't judge, but offered her love and support.

I sent Dickie a letter, and a copy of an essay I had written about my mother. Then I decided to write another essay. I started writing an essay about Dickie, to let him know how much he had meant to me over the years. The process of remembering, of writing about our adventures, made me feel better. I wanted to document the experiences we had shared over the years and tell him how much I loved him. It took me several days and eight pages to finish my memoir. I vowed to take the essay with me when I went to Harrisburg. I prayed he would still be alive when I got there.

When I got to western Pennsylvania, my joy at seeing my friends and relatives was overshadowed by my concern for Dickie. Shopping with my best friend and dinner with my former coworkers was fun, but I still couldn't get Dickie out of my mind. Even my twentieth high school reunion wasn't as much fun as earlier reunions had been. I laughed and talked with friends I had grown up with, but my heart wasn't in it. My heart was miles away, in Harrisburg with Dickie.

The afternoon after the reunion, I went over to my friend Kathy's house. I asked her if I could make a long distance call. She nodded and stood nearby, as she knew I was calling Dickie.

"Hello? Who is this?" Dickie's voice was barely recognizable. His voice has always been deep, with a melodic quality to it, reflecting his training in opera and classical music. The voice that answered the phone was weak and distant.

"It's Marvella, Dickie." I tried to sound lighthearted. I didn't want him to sense the shock I felt when I heard his voice.

"Oh, Marvella. It's nice to hear from you." He sounded strange, as if his mind was somewhere else.

"I'm in Pittsburgh. I'm coming to Harrisburg to visit you tomorrow. I rented a car, so I should be there in the late afternoon."

"What?" He did not seem to understand. He was silent for a few seconds. Then he said, "You better come to see me before I die."

The emphasis he gave to that last word sent a chill through me, even though it was hot in Kathy's apartment.

I didn't know how to answer him, which didn't matter because then he started to talk about his fur coat. I hung up the phone with trepidation, because I knew that the person I would see the next day would not be the Dickie I had known for so many years.

I started out on the Pennsylvania Turnpike with a heavy heart. It was a beautiful, summer day, but I did not enjoy it. I used to love to drive across Pennsylvania, looking at the small farms and towns of my home state. But this time, I didn't even notice the scenery. It took all of my strength just to keep the car on the road. I willed myself not to think too much, as my eyes would blur with tears. Four hours felt like four days.

But as much as I tried to control my thoughts and emotions, I still thought about him. Would he recognize me? When I was a little girl, my mother developed dementia. It could have been Alzheimer's disease, but no one knew about that in the late sixties. I used to follow her down the street, trying to convince her to return home with me. Sometimes she didn't even know I was her daughter. Would I have to go through that with Dickie? What would he look like? Would he look anything like the chocolate colored man who always looked so good in designer suits? And if he didn't, would I be able to handle it? I didn't want to cry in front of him.

I used to enjoy driving through the many tunnels that were part of the Turnpike system. But now the moments of darkness seem to reflect my worse fears. The Allegheny Mountain Tunnel, the Tuscarora Mountain Tunnel, the Kittatinny

Mountain Tunnel and the Blue Mountain Tunnel—each one brought me closer to Harrisburg. When I got off at the Carlisle exit, my hands were shaking. I wanted to see Dickie, but I didn't know if I wanted to see him bedridden. Maybe I should have stayed away. Maybe it would have been better to remember him like he was the last time that I saw him. But it's too late for that now, I thought as I drove into Harrisburg.

When I got to the house, Dickie's mother Rose, who had recently had a stroke rendering her unable to talk, greeted me. She gave me a smile and a kiss. Dickie's sister Carolyn looked tired and haggard due to the pressure of caring for her older brother and mother while working full-time as a Department of Social Services supervisor. Rose pointed towards the stairs. Dickie was bedridden on the second floor, in a room that had previously been used as the "television room." On my last visit, Dickie and I had watched a movie together in that room.

I went up the steps slowly, trying to delay the inevitable. I was shocked when I entered the room and saw Dickie. The person in the bed was a frail, skeletal figure, with gray hair, dark mottled skin and sunken eyes. When he saw me, a sparkle entered his eyes, and his parched lips stretched into a smile.

"Marvella! You made it!" A slight lilt came into his voice as he called my name and reached out to hug me.

As I put my arms around him, I could feel only a thin layer of skin stretched over bones. I was afraid to hug him too tightly. He seemed so fragile. Neither of my parents had reached such an emaciated state before they died.

I was afraid to kiss him. I had read about AIDS, and how it was transmitted, but I couldn't control the reflex that caused me to break contact with him. I hated myself for it and I prayed that he hadn't noticed.

There was a nursing aide in the room with him. She nodded at me when I came in. "Hello. I'm Mrs. Adams."

I smiled shakily. "I'm Marvella."

"It's so nice that you came all the way from California to visit your cousin."

"Yeah." I didn't know what else to say. I didn't feel nice.

When I sat in a chair next to him, Mrs. Adams went over to Dickie's bedside.

"Dickie?" She had a Bible in her hands. "Would you like to have prayer since your Cousin Marvella is here?" she asked.

"NO!" he said vehemently.

I was surprised, as Dickie had always been very religious.

She looked at me for help, but I had nothing to say. Dickie had been the religious one, not me.

"But Dickie, I'm an ordained minister," she said in a soft voice.

He looked at her with anger in his eyes. "I don't care. You aren't my personal pastor."

She looked at me again. I could hear Rose and Carolyn coming up the stairs.

She looked toward the door. "Well, maybe I could have prayer with your family?"

He looked over at Rose and Carolyn as they came into the room. "Sure, if you want to."

Rose, Carolyn and I gathered around Dickie's hospital bed and joined Mrs. Adams in a prayer. Then we went back downstairs, leaving Dickie alone with the television. Mrs. Adams was leaving for the day. After she left, Carolyn came into the kitchen to talk to me.

Her dark eyes darted toward the ceiling.

"How is he doing?" I asked, afraid of her answer.

She shook her head. "He is taking so much medicine. Some of those pills are causing him to have hallucinations. He just goes in and out of his head. Sometimes he is okay, sometimes he talks to people who aren't there."

I looked at the steps. "I understand. I think I will go back up and sit with him for awhile."

She nodded and went to fix dinner for Rose. I went back upstairs and sat with him for several hours.

He pointed to the chair. "Sit down. We will go out to dinner in a little while. Where do you want to go?"

I held back tears, because I knew that we would never go out to dinner again. "I don't know. You pick." I tried to go along with his conversation, just like I did with my mother when I was twelve.

He pulled at his hair. "Look at this grey hair. I need to dye it. What do you think?" Dickie had always been very particular about his appearance.

"I guess so," I answered, even though I knew that a bottle of Grecian Formula would not change the way he looked.

He started talking to persons that were not in the room, inviting them to sit down, in his usual gracious manner. I sat next to him and listened. He seemed to have forgotten I was even in the room. I wondered if he was doing like Momma had done, talking to people that had died years ago.

I heard a scraping. I looked under the bed. Dickie's devoted little dog was lying there, guarding his master. Rose came in and shooed the dog from the room. A few minutes later he was back, seeking comfort from his friend of many years. The dog looked so sad and lost. He didn't know why his fun loving master couldn't get up and play with him any more. I commiserated with him. "I wanted the old Dickie back, too."

Carolyn was going out to get something to eat. She asked me if I wanted to go along. Dickie was still talking to imaginary visitors, so I left the room and went downstairs to join her. She drove to a local supermarket and picked up a few things.

I had never been around Carolyn that much in all of my visits to Harrisburg, Baltimore, and Washington, D.C. This was probably the first time that we had ever been alone. We did have something in common, as both of us had worked for the state welfare department. She asked me about my life. I gave her simple answers. I didn't feel comfortable with her.

"I don't know how you can live out there," she said.

I shrugged. "It's okay."

We were nearing the house. I could see the light on upstairs in Dickie's room. Carolyn maneuvered the car into the driveway. "I like Oakland. But I don't like San Francisco. Too many faggots."

I gripped the bottom of my seat to keep from hitting her. My jaw clinched, but it was too dark for her to see and I doubted if she would have noticed anyway. We got out of the car with the groceries.

I wanted to say something, but I could not open my mouth. I looked up at the window again. Carolyn's beloved brother, her only sibling, was lying a few feet away dying, and she had the nerve to talk about "faggots"? No wonder Dickie had spent the last thirty years living a double life.

As I walked behind Carolyn toward the back door, I knew that I no longer liked her. I no longer respected her. She was just a relative, a person that I was connected to because I had been adopted thirty-seven years ago.

After eating quickly and in relative silence, I went back upstairs to sit with the only person in this house I really cared about. Dickie was more lucid now. He talked about reducing his medication to clear his mind. We sat together for several hours. It was hard to look at him. But I was thankful that he was still breathing, still fighting. Then I left to go to bed, too emotionally drained to sit with him any longer.

I went upstairs to the third floor, to Dickie's old room. I looked around at all of the things that filled his cluttered room. All that he had left from a lifetime of accomplishment and adventure was jumbled together in this small room tucked under the roof.

After his mother had suffered a stroke, he had given up everything to move from Washington back to Harrisburg to take care of her. He probably never dreamed that she would end up trying to take care of him. I picked up an old passport from 1960 that was lying on the dresser. I looked at all of the Central and South American stamps and at the picture of a twenty-one-year-old Dickie. Dickie had always loved to travel and had been all over the world. He had a tiny Casio keyboard sitting on a sofa, a small cry from the beautiful grand piano he had once possessed in Baltimore.

The room smelled like Paco Rabanne, Dickie's favorite cologne. I used to smell it all of the time when I stayed in his bedroom at his Baltimore and D.C. homes. Dickie had always relegated the television to his bedroom. When I visited him, I would stay in his bedroom watching television while he was at work. There was a television in this room too. I turned it on and watched it for a while until I fell asleep, comforted by Dickie's scent.

The next morning, when I passed Dickie's room to go to the bathroom, I glanced into the room. He was getting off of the portable toilet. Before I could turn my head, I noticed his withered flanks. He looked like a starving refugee from Somalia or a concentration camp survivor from Auschwitz, not my beloved cousin. How could this disease do this to him? I hurried into the bathroom and splashed water on my face before I started crying again.

When I went back upstairs to dress, I heard Rose come up the steps. When I went down to the second floor again, she was dragging the container of waste towards the bathroom. I panicked, as the waste was sloshing around in the bucket, threatening to spill over her, as she didn't have the strength to lift it. I was scared, as I knew the virus could be spread by direct contact with bodily fluids.

"No, Rose!" I screamed. "Leave it alone. Leave it for the nurse to empty."

She continued to drag the container, grunting and shaking her head. Dickie was her son; she was supposed to be able to take care of him when he was sick, just like when he was a little boy.

I was sweating. I didn't want to handle the container either. I didn't know where the nurse had left the rubber gloves. I was afraid of touching the waste. Maybe I had an open sore on my hands that I wasn't aware of. Maybe I could get AIDS from emptying a slop jar. I hated myself for the wild thoughts that I couldn't control.

There was a knock on the front door. It had to be Mrs. Adams. I ran downstairs and opened the door, then explained what was going on. She came upstairs and explained to Rose that she shouldn't handle the containers. I felt faint. I was upset, both by Rose's actions and my reaction. I went downstairs to get breakfast. In a few minutes, Rose came down also.

Soon I could hear Dickie talking and laughing with Mrs. Adams. I ate in silence while Rose watched. I had always liked Cousin Rose, but we had never been close. I had always liked her sister, Cousin Mag, better. Mag had been the liaison between my adopted mother and my birth mother, so we had always had a special connection. Mag had died last year. But Rose reminded me of my mother in some ways. The soft clipped accent she had shared with my mother was now replaced by snorts and grunts, the only sounds she could make. She tried to communicate with her eyes when her sounds failed, but it was still hard for me to talk to her.

After a few minutes, I went to sit with Dickie while he ate breakfast. He could only take small bites of his sandwich and small sips of his soda. A sandwich that could have been consumed in a few minutes took him over a half an hour to finish. I stared at the television. While he ate, his dog came back in the room. Dickie gave bits of the sandwich to his friend.

After he ate, he handed me a pad and pen. He pointed at the bottles of pills that covered the table next to the bed. "Write down all of the names on these bottles."

There were at least ten bottles. I picked up each bottle, recited its name, and wrote it on the notepad. He nodded his head. This was Dickie the nurse in action.

"One of these is making me hallucinate. I'm going to call my doctor and find out which one it is."

After I finished, I handed the paper back to him.

We sat for a few hours, watching television. Then, Carolyn's daughter Tina called, asking me to go to lunch with her. I got ready to leave. I promised Dickie I would spend the rest of the day with him when I returned.

When I got back to the house later that afternoon, Dickie was alert. He must have eliminated the drug that was affecting his hold on reality.

The television was on and I sat down next to him. I told him about my third trip to London the previous year.

He smiled and listened intently.

"Remember when I was here two years ago? You were planning to go to Egypt."

He started crying. "I'll never get to go now. Why me? There is so much that I want to do!"

I had no answer. I stared blankly at the television.

"You know I have been diagnosed with cancer. It is attacking my insides."

I still didn't answer. I wanted him to know he didn't have to lie to me. I wanted him to know that Bonita had already told me the truth. But I couldn't speak. Why did he feel that he had to lie to me?

The news was on television. The reporter was talking about the AIDS epidemic. My breath caught, but still I didn't say anything.

"What do you think about AIDS?" he asked.

"I think that it is horrible. It is a terrible disease. I think that more research needs to be done on its causes and how to prevent it." I know, Dickie, I know, I thought to myself.

Dickie became silent. He looked over at me. "Why are people so concerned with other people's sexuality?" He waited for my answer.

"I think that it is so stupid. People have no right to judge anyone else's lifestyle. I could care less who other people go to bed with. As long as they are happy, that's all that matters." I looked at Dickie. He seemed satisfied with my answer.

I was surprised by the question. Dickie's family had never acknowledged his homosexuality, and his lifestyle was never discussed.

I had brought some essays of mine for him, but he could no longer read. His sight was failing. We talked about my writing, and I read one of my essays to him. Since he tired easily, I decided to wait until the next day to read him the story of our lives together.

I had an appointment the next morning, and when I got back to the house, Dickie was asleep. I waited several hours, but then I had to leave, as I didn't want to drive on the turnpike at night.

Before I left, I made a videotape of Dickie's room on the third floor, because I knew that I would never see it again filled with Dickie's aura. I found the musical score of "La Boheme," an opera Dickie had performed in the previous year with the local Civic Light Opera Company. Dickie had highlighted his part, and had written in his stage directions. I put the score in my bag, as a memento of Dickie's lifelong love of opera.

He was still asleep when I left, and I knew that I would never see him alive again. When I got back to Pittsburgh, I called him to tell him I made it back safely.

I regretted the fact that I never got the chance to read my essay to him.

After I got back home to California, I wondered daily about Dickie's condition. I couldn't afford to make any long distance calls, so I hoped my cousins would keep me informed of any changes. I sent a copy of my essay about Dickie to my cousin Norva in Baltimore, Bonita's sister. I asked her to read it to Dickie when she went to visit him. I had brought a lot of old snapshots from Pennsylvania, and I looked at my pictures of Dickie taken during my many visits.

On the evening of September 19, 1994, I received a call from Bonita.

"Dickie's gone," she said. "He died around 4 PM this afternoon. We all drove up from Baltimore yesterday to see him. He was in the hospital. Norva read your essay to him."

"I'm glad that he got to hear it."

"Well, she had to leave out the part about him being gay because Rose was in the room."

I didn't respond.

"He couldn't talk by then, but he could still understand it. He smiled when she read the funny parts. He cried some too."

We talked a few more minutes about our memories of Dickie, and about his love of music. I couldn't afford to come back to Pennsylvania, but I got the funeral information so I could send flowers. When I got off of the phone, I sat down on my bed and started crying in loud, heaving sobs. I felt like a part of my heart had died with him.

I thought about what Bonita had said. I was glad Dickie had died knowing how much he had meant to me. I was annoyed that Norva had edited the essay, as I felt Dickie needed to know that someone in his family approved of him no matter what kind of lifestyle he had led. I only hoped that our talk before his death had eased his mind. I wished I had talked to him about his lifestyle and his disease when he had asked me those questions. I wonder if he had asked me those questions because he wanted to discuss his sexuality. I will never know the answer to that question.

He was gone. My Dickie was gone. My champion, my defender, my Capricorn soul brother was gone from this earth. I wanted to scream, I wanted to hurt someone and make them hurt as much as I did. I felt helpless and alone. I wanted to crawl in a dark hole and be alone with my memories of Dickie.

I pulled out the old birthday and Christmas cards that I had received from him and touched the writing. I looked at pictures of him, so young, so happy and so full of life. I wanted to kill the person that had given him the disease that had taken him from me. Maybe he was already dead.

Dickie has been gone fifteen years now. There will always be a hollow place in my heart that will never be filled. There have been so many things over the years I wish I could have shared with him. I especially missed his presence when I received my MFA degree in December 2004. I keep his picture on a table in my living room, next to the pictures of my deceased parents and other long gone relatives. On the same table, I keep the candle I carried when I participated in a candlelight vigil on World AIDS Day a few years ago.

There have been so many advances in AIDS medications since his death. I wish he could have had some of those medicines available to him. And after all this time, I'm still angry. I'm angry he could not have lived his life openly and proudly and have been accepted by his family. I'm still angry with my cousins, who perpetuated a heterosexual myth and forced Dickie to live a dual life. I'm angry that my good, kind, wonderful cousin was robbed of his life after only fifty-three short years. I am angry at the disease called AIDS, which stole the only relative that believed in me and encouraged my creativity.

AIDS has changed my life forever. I haven't seen my cousins since Dickie's death, but I have talked to them on the telephone. A few years ago, Rose died. Even though so many years have passed since Dickie left us, I still harbor resentment towards them. I can't imagine visiting Baltimore, Washington or Harrisburg without Dickie being there.

But beyond the anger, there is the knowledge that Dickie is still with me. In my mind, I can see the charming, handsome man with the twinkle in his eyes and the welcoming smile. I still remember his laugh and that scent. In Spring 2009, "Fabulous," a poem I wrote about him was published in an anthology. A little part of him will live on in each person that reads my poem.

Sometimes, I dream about him and wake up to the faint smell of Paco. I hope he forgave me for not telling him how I felt about his homosexuality. I hope he forgave all of us. And I hope he knew the answers to those questions I never really answered.

The Closeness of Strangers

Michael Boccardo

I knew the chance was slim. One year with no warnings,
not even a lesion on the back or neck, surfacing like some coffee stain

along the crease of a tablecloth. As the nurse siphons
my blood, I hear the crack of t-cells colliding like billiard balls, blind

in their habits, a dizzy traffic jam of crimson caught inside
a slender tube. You have good veins, she says, the way an English professor

praises composition but criticizes careless regard for grammar.
I know it's her way, a distraction from the needle buried

in the pale meat of what may soon grow spoiled. But I can't help
sculpting another life from the portraits beside us, the Crayola sketches

scotch-taped to her walls, names like Nancy and Erin and Isaac
as bold as the yellow oval of sun suspended midair, a life

where the closeness of strangers hooks her body tighter to the chain
of her husband's, their arms and legs locked, fingers braided like links

in a fence. The same hands that smooth a bandage into place, then
catalogue my life alongside others, glass houses, neighbors all—
never touching.

Jay

Nagueyalti Warren

I. Jay: A Trilogy

Mamma says the worst has happened. It's morning and daddy is fixing
his eggs in the little black skillet. Mamma's eyes are red and swollen.

She has not combed her hair. She looks like she doesn't care.
Frying eggs spit grease on the chrome stove. Daddy's jaw is set.

His ears go back. *Deserved it,* daddy says. *Damned son-of-a-bitch!*
Mamma drops her juice glass, crashing, blue splinters on the floor.

That's my child you talking 'bout. My son, and I ain't no bitch you
son-of-a-bastard. They don't see me standing near the toaster in my

flannel teddy bear jammies granny sent. I'm shaking and start to cry.
Boy made his bed hard, now he got to lie in it, daddy turns from the sink,

pops pepper on his eggs. *Jimmy that's your son you talking 'bout.*
He ain't in the damn bed by himself. We in it too. We all affected.

Mamma's crying, her nose dripping. *The hell you say.* Daddy's temple
veins thump on his head. Mamma sobs, *It's a death sentence. It shouldn't be*

a death sentence. Daddy slams down his fork, *he sinned.* Mamma shouts,
we sinned too, but we didn't die. We just got pregnant and got married.

Is Jay dying? My voice shakes and they both jump and turn around to me.
James died a long time ago, daddy mumbles, but mamma sighs and she

pulls me to her coffee breath, *he's sick baby.* I'm seven, my big brother
is nineteen and daddy says he cannot come home and mamma says we

are going to get him and bring him home and daddy can take his ratty ass
and go straight to hell. We take the Greyhound to San Francisco through

that gate that isn't even golden but red, red as blood Jay spits when he tries
to eat, like red snot running from his nose when I give him pepper pot soup.

Daddy stays in the house but will not talk to Jay. Mamma says pay him no mind.
Jay's tears slide from his long black lashes. They look like jewels on his face.

His cracked lips do not smile and he can't sing songs off the radio, not even
Rapper's Delight. At night he sweats. I wipe his face with my Cyndi Lauper

cloth until mamma makes me go to bed. I pray that Jay won't die because he is gay.
Daddy says all gay men die and go to hell. Happy shouldn't kill. I think
heaven is the happy place.

Maybe I'm confused like when I thought the wafer was the white skin
of Jesus and refused to eat it.

The last day of school I come home to see Jay loaded into an orange and white
ambulance, red top rolling round, doors slam, and it screeches away down Imperial

Highway. Mamma crying, daddy holding her up but she sees me and grabs my hand.
Get my keys. I'm going with my baby. Come on, mamma says.

Daddy won't come. *You old stubborn fool! May your soul rot in your pious shit.* Mamma backs out the truck and we follow the siren's whine to the emergency room door.

Mamma running almost falls but I catch her arm and we have to wait for Jay to get a room and daddy comes and we are waiting and Jay's friend Jerome comes.

Daddy jumps up and socks him in the mouth knocking out his front teeth and blood and the police take daddy away and Jerome is crying and mamma is crying and I am crying

and Jay slips away at eight fifty two p.m. when it just starts to rain and lightning streaks the hospital windows, thunder rumbles, drowning out my mamma's screams.

...

II In the Eighties, My Son Jay

He looks me dead in my face, my man face and tell me he don't like girls
except to be his good friends, hang out in the mall and all. I'm not seeing

what he means, not knowing what the hell he is saying to me, his daddy.
Him smiling, looking like a cat what swallowed the mouse, licking his lips.

He say dad I'm homosexual. I hit the wall with me fist. Bust hole, a man hole.
I taught you to be a man. He steps back saying, it's just me dad. I am just what

I am. Out my house. No nasty shit in here. Okay he says quiet. Hurt catch
on the turn of his thick lips. He looks past me, liquid brown eyes full of regret.

My throat dry. My hands sweat. I feel tears freeze in the top of my throat.
Why my son? What I do? What I don't do? What I can do? Heavenly Father!

He goes down the back steps, his mamma staring at me, telling me to stop him,
but I'm the one sending him away from here—away from everyone who knows

me. I'm done with it two years when my wife come waking me up with that
phone call saying he sick to death. He can't bring that sickness up in here.

She curse me. Brings him anyway. What a man can do? Woman/mamma crazy
wild about her child. She spoil him up, she the one make him weak, she the one.

So I bear the shame. Disease without a name I tell my friends and they don't pry.
My son, six-foot one, ninety-nine pounds. I pray. I cry. Then I wait for him to
die.

III My Son Jay, In The Eighties

He was a gorgeous baby, so lovely I had to always dress him in blue
or people would take him for a girl, thick hair curled around his oval
face, almond eyes with lashes thick and black, his cupid lips smiling
whenever he saw me. He walked early, talked before he could walk.
Named him James Harrison Walker, after his daddy, but Jimmy wouldn't
let me call him Little Jimmy. We agreed on Jay who grew so big and tall.
He was a perfect boy, so easy to love, so talented, artistic, and perceptive.
His father was angry when Jay came out the closet, but I wasn't caught
off guard. I didn't want him to be any kind of macho man. He was love.
A man who would not even kill a fly or stomp and ant. He just wanted
to be free, was so much like me, flesh of my flesh, bone of my bone.
Now he is gone. Just wanted to express himself like anybody else.
His own daddy made him feel like his life and love were wrong, like a
man can be only be one thing, but my Jay was so fly—my mariposa.

the gravedigger

Clara Nura Sala

for Beer Musandirire: city gravedigger, AIDS epidemic;
Harare, Zimbabwe

7
is
a
holy
number

7
holds a
beginning
&
end

I dig 7 days a week
& the bodies never stop
behind their tribal masks
the dead grow younger
our ancestors shuffling backward
to no future

with no condoms
faithless husbands
press into frightened wives
&
my eyes never close

in shallow sleep
I dream
of scraping and dust
I dream
of washing my hands
over
&
over
I hammer two branches of Acacia*
into
one
cross
two
three
a miracle

they multiply across the fields
      until they are a cloud of single-celled locusts
      the death rattle
      in our
         mothers
          fathers

      sons
      daughters
      our grandchildren's eyes withered brown nipples
            swim in red milk

      even as my
      eyelids
      droop

trapping dead spirits in my pupils
their skinny hands
grip
my
shovel
when the
handle
snaps
we dig with our fingers
at the end of 7 days

we start again

**Acacia: graceful, sturdy tree found in parts of Africa and the Middle East*

Punch Line

Keith Wilson

God's script
scrawled into mountains,
his jokes
coded in lowercase,
punctuated
in my uncle's blood

a notebook's fluttering
pages, a dozen
unfinished thoughts,
a punch line
too small
to be target of
my hatred

Web of Life

Roopali Kambo

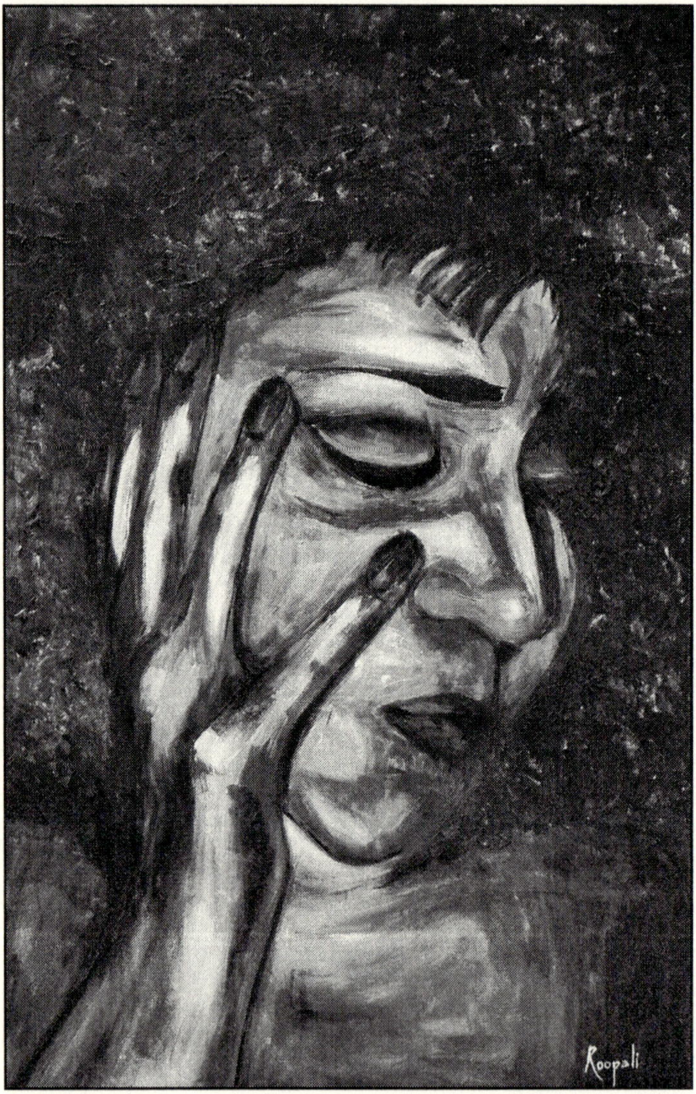

SECTION III

LIVE ONE MORE DAY

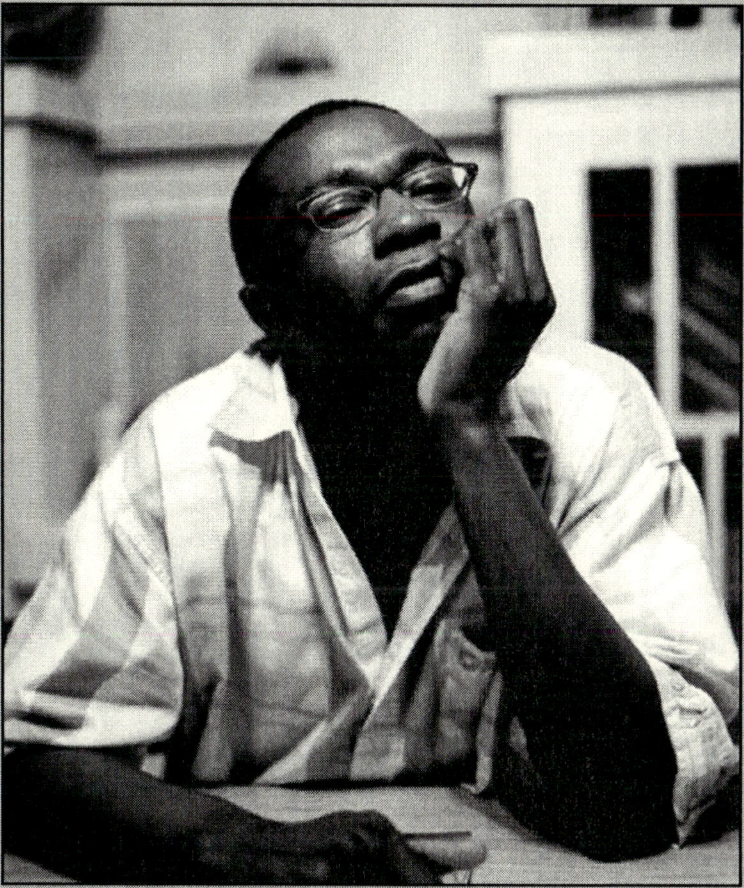

UNTITLED | **Viet Lê**

Cielo

Emanuel Xavier

for Joe Jimenez

Lover with the distance of a star
on a clear night
I will always find you
in the same space
helping me find my calling
while huddled on rooftops
imagining you shine for me alone

When you said you wanted to drive across the border
introduce me to all your cousins
so they could watch us fall in love
know this—I would've held your hand all the way to Mexico

I would've swallowed all your demons with my kisses
What I saw *en tus ojos* is that luxury is not a precious stone
It is reading the most beautiful poetry etched on skin
dreaming of someday nestling this scarred head
on your tattooed shoulder

Like the sky above, I want to span the spaces between us
from Bushwick to Aztlan
I want to take you to the projects of Coney Island
where I first lost my innocence
because with you I have newfound morality
I want to go with you to that alley

where your nightmares began
unfold your heart and crawl inside
to always carry me within your soul
I want to take you to the piers
where I learned to survive
look out into the Hudson River
and pray thanks to all the drowned divas
I want to be your Rio Grande and guide you safely over to freedom
and the innocent smiles of children hungering for inspiration
I want to bathe you in spiritual waters and light candles
to the mistress of death
tenderly caressing *tu corazón y tu cuerpo*
with these lips smoothed by Chap Stick
With you, I want to enjoy everything from *cuchifrito*
to *chile con papa y nopal*
I want to show you the *barrio* where I grew up
and was eventually nearly killed
Grateful I'm still here with the opportunity
of someday holding you in my arms

Looking out to the moon we both share,
I answer these questions—
The best laugh I ever had
was probably provoked by the bratty little boy in me
The most transformative truth I ever told
was called "Deliverance"
The person who has hurt me the most in life
is the one I likely resemble
It is the reason I both fear and desire fatherhood

how I wish I could say you were my first
how I would have wanted to be your sun
warming that lovely brown skin
I will hold on to this memory and the fading sound of your voice

maybe you never got to read my poem
maybe we are living on borrowed time
maybe I was too late to be the one
maybe I am not the one
to come between this rude religion of relationship
but still
we fight this revolution
together
underneath the same sky

When you feel a breeze
remember
mi cielo
remember

I'll wait for the courage of your *promesas*
I'll wait for you until our day has come

Ode to an AIDS Survivor

Victor Pond

Even when the darkness bends
extruding the light
leaving behind an intangible night
....
there you will be
silently defiant
unmindful of the void before you
knowing that tomorrow
the sun will rise
to swallow up the shadow.
....
With the confidence
of Griots....the ones who taste stories
before sharing them.....You will walk
leaving behind carved memories
so strangers behind you
will burn with the desire
to live one more day.

The Visit

Reginald Harris

We were on the other side of town anyway, visiting his family, when we said to ourselves, *Why don't we stop by to see Kraig's mother?* It had been about a year since we'd seen Valerie. Although we had called to see how she was doing and had sent her a Christmas card, we thought it would be good to put in an appearance, to actually see how she was, to let her know that we were still around and thinking of her. We called first, of course, since she's so often in the streets or out of town. She was home, said she was on her way out somewhere, but had the time to see us before she had to leave.

Her little street was just beginning to toss off the thick blanket of snow thrown on it from the last storm. It was passable but still not completely cleared, and Valerie's neighbors were clearing sidewalks and digging out their cars. The walk leading up to her house was still snow-covered, although packed down.

Valerie greeted us with hugs and kisses and saying things like, "you all keep putting on weight," the usual mother stuff. Her paneled living room was warm and seemed unchanged from the way it was when Kraig, his sister, brother, and I were growing up. We all used to congregate here before heading into the streets and trouble. The TV was on but muted, like a hand had covered its mouth, while darkness leaked down from the quiet upstairs of the two-story house. Kraig's mother seemed unchanged, too, still bright and cheerful, despite all we had put her through back then and now. She also hadn't grown any since then, either, and we towered over her as she continued to hold us.

We asked Valerie about her front walk and she said she hadn't gotten one of the neighbor kids to clean it off yet. Since it snowed ever other day lately, why bother? We offered to do it for her, the least we could do really and grabbed the two shovels she had already set just inside the front door before she could protest too much (although, come to think of it, there really wasn't a lot of protesting, nor did we think it odd that there just happened to be a pair of shovels at the ready when we arrived).

We acted quickly to remove the snow. It had suddenly warmed up, so it was softer and easier to manage than the stuff we'd had to dig ourselves out of in front of our own place. The top layer came up easily once we got into a rhythm, the shovels singing in counterpoint to those of Valerie's neighbors. We each started at a different end of the walk and met in the middle, the *shhh/thunk, shhh/thunk* of our work sounding more like we were digging a hole than clearing snow. Every now and then one of us would take a break, stopping and looking around as if waiting for something or looking for someone to come out and help us.

But there was no one, so we went back to work. One of us banged the heavier of the two shovels into the hard packed ice under the soft outer covering, breaking it up to allow the other to slide under it and toss it to the side. We'd been told to leave the car wrapped in ice, since Valerie had no intention of driving, but figured, since we were out there anyway . . . And so we chopped and scraped and sweated and cursed ourselves for not listening to the woman, until we had cleaned off the car and made a pretty good exit path for her small car. Then, sprinkling kitty litter instead of bread crumbs behind us, we backed our way up the front walk, up the three damp steps, and into the house, where we immediately got yelled at for not wiping our feet before coming inside.

After scraping our soles on the doorstep and putting the shovels away, we took off our coats, sat down in the living room, and caught ourselves up on our lives. Valerie was glad to hear that I was going back to school; my other half talked about his new security job, when not hypnotized by NCAA March Madness on the large color TV set. The two of us glanced around the room and up the darkened stairs then asked Valerie about her life. She sighed deeply.

"Well, you know Karl is in the hospital now. There's a problem with his heart. That comes from his family." She pointed at me as I nodded. "A lot of you have heart problems. Karl's got a weak valve and an infection too, so they really can't do anything to help him until the infection clears up. And Ada just came out of the hospital. She went in to have one of her ovaries removed and while she was there the doctors took a look at the other one and said that one had to come out, too. So she was in the hospital for a long time. She's going back in next week to have them take a look at this lump in her breast. She had one taken out on the left side a few years ago, it was benign, and now she found another on the right side."

Valerie shook her head.

"It's been rough, it's been rough."

The cheering and yelling from the basketball game seemed ghoulish and loud. We both looked at this tiny woman, always so helpful to everyone else. Our eyes washed around the room, the tables, the mantles, and piano filled with pictures of her children and grandchildren, nieces and nephews, her late husband, and extended family.

"But how are you doing?" we asked.

"I guess I'm okay." She sighed.

"Ada said there really was nothing I could do for her while she was in the hospital, so I went up to Ohio to visit my brother and his family, just to get away, since I knew I'd have to look after her when she got out. My neighbors come and take me to the hospital since I'm not going to drive in all this ice and snow. So I get to go to the market and see Karl. People come to see me, like you two, which is good, and Ada brings her kids and the grandbabies over too, or I go over to see them. It's rough sometimes, but I manage. What else am I going to do? You do what you have to."

She nodded her head. "I'm all right."

There was nothing more to say. Valerie had to go to the hospital before it got too late. She'd already arranged for her neighbor to take her and so didn't accept our offer to drive her. She asked about our respective families, said she hadn't heard from mine in a while, which was no surprise since they seldom talk to me anymore either.

"You two should come to see me more often, sometimes when I have more time," she said as the three of us rose from our seats.

"Don't be strangers."

"We will, we will," we said. We won't, we won't.

Then, in that awkward moment of silence right before we left, I had to be the one to say what all of us were thinking.

"I keep wanting to go upstairs and see Kraig. I'm sorry... I'm sorry, but . . . he's here, I can feel it. He's still here, and I keep thinking . . . " I paused, uncertain if I should go on. "I know it's been over a year, and you've got enough to deal with right now, but I keep *waiting* for him, waiting to see him walk in that door any minute now."

And so we stood there, all three of us in our coats, a hugging knot in the middle of the living room, surrounded by family portraits, crying and sniffling, my partner and I tightly holding hands as Valerie murmured softly, "Be well, be careful, be *CARE*-full" into our chests. We held each other, holding on, rocking, somehow all of us still holding on, until her neighbor rang the bell, and it was time for Kraig's mother to visit her child in the hospital again.

Quest

Basanta Kar

A quest for thirteen years
mitigates at his arms crossed
warm bosom, the sounds of silence
work in tandem
I trample the virus
stem blooms a new bud.

Lost love was for me
this love is for him.
Still a mother's soul laments
terrible is this exile self imposed.

He is positive, I am positive
look for a life perennially negative
re-beginning new colostrums feeding
amidst amplifying networks of fellow positives
I imagine a line parallel horizontal
in the land undulated
forget the lines zigzag, vertical, linear.
Early monsoon flattens the *Gomti*
I enjoy night and day
compose poetry out of page.

(A thirty-four year old divorcee HIV positive woman married to a HIV positive man. She is from Lucknow, Uttar Pradesh, India)

Dancing in My Dreams

Ran Walker

The city was just as I had remembered it in my dreams.

The taxi drifted serenely up the West Side Highway, sailing past the silhouetted skyline that had once been our playground. As I caught a view of the Hudson River glimmering from the reflections of a million lights rippling across its surface, I could see Serena's face. I could feel its warmth against my fingers as I pulled her into our last kiss that November day three years ago. Her perfume still tickled my nostrils like a phantom haunting me in the most delicious sense of the word.

There was no acceptable explanation for why I had left. Sure there was the opportunity to study on the West Coast, but love should have made me unpack my bags. Her tears alone should have forced me to defer for at least another year—just until she could get her own situation worked out. But my own dreams called out in voices so strong that I could hear nothing else.

She had begged me not to go; I had asked her to come. When she refused to accept my invitation, I took it personally, and from there our relationship disintegrated. Our love, once a ripe fruit bubbling with the sweetest nectar I had ever tasted, withered slowly on the vine from neglect.

Why I had chosen to pack a bag and fly across the country late in the evening to see her wasn't even all that apparent to me. All I knew was that I had to let her know that I didn't want to move forward in this life without her by my side. I had no specific idea of what I would do next if she were to commit herself once again to our love, but I was prepared to stay in New York until we were able to figure that out.

The e-mails had been short and sweet, reminiscent of the way things were when we were together. She said that she missed me, that she still loved me. I told her that I had made the ultimate mistake when I left her. Even her melodic voice over the phone soothed the ache of regret I had come to know in the solitude of her absence.

"We can try again," I stated emphatically in our last conversation.

"But you're there. And I'm here," was her response.

I didn't know if that was an excuse or an invitation.

And now, in the depth of the evening, I was seated in the back of a taxicab headed to Harlem, a solitary duffle bag resting beside me and a heart full to capacity of a love that refused to die amidst the trials of three years.

I imagined her as she appeared in the pictures she e-mailed me: her hair short and naturally curly, her eyes wide with tenderness, her smile framed by dimples, her teeth like glistening pearls, her skin a flawless sheet of silk dipped in caramel and draped around an exquisite and well-formed frame. How could I have ever walked away from her?

The taxi eased into her neighborhood, a neighborhood in which I had spent many nights intoxicated from our lovemaking (only to stumble back onto the train in the morning and barely make it to work on time). With the reflection of the street lamps against the brownstone, I felt as if I were gazing upon a castle, and inside that castle was the woman fate had revealed to be my queen.

Moments after I pushed the buzzer, the intercom rang to life with her sleepy voice.

"Serena, it's me. Kyle," I said.

"Kyle? Oh my god!"

Over the intercom I could hear her shuffling things around and then the door buzzed and unlocked, allowing me entrance.

The building hadn't changed much, but my mind registered every picture on the walls as something brand new. Reaching for the handrail, I ascended the stairs slowly, unsure of what her reaction to my presence would be.

I was prepared for anything. If there was someone in there with her, I would just deal with the situation as best I could. I had come prepared to win this woman's heart, and if it meant I had to confront someone else to get my point across, that was just the cost of following my heart.

She was already standing in the doorway looking very surprised when I reached the top of the stairs. Dressed only in a white ribbed tank top and a pair of tight jeans, she embraced me excitedly. For a moment all I could do was hold her, squeeze her, as if I was trying to absorb three years of lost warmth from her. She snuggled into my embrace and held on as if she shared my sentiment.

"I missed you so much," I said. "I had to see you."

"I missed you, too," she responded.

After what seemed like one beautiful, interminable moment, she released my body and took me by the hand, guiding me into her dimly lit apartment, the only lighting coming from night lights placed strategically throughout her apartment and a solitary lamp resting on a coffee table in her living room.

"What are you doing here?" she asked, still registering my presence in New York.

"After our last conversation, I had to come here to let you know that I am real about how I feel."

"And you couldn't have told me over the phone?"

My eyebrow lifted involuntarily as if I had just been swatted across the face with a thin white glove. I replayed her question in my mind, searching desperately for some semblance of humor beyond the words, only to find that the words lay bare.

"Did I miss something?" I asked.

She stood up, and without answering my question, offered me a drink. I accepted a Smirnoff Ice, but a sip from the cool beverage did little in the way of easing my nervousness.

"It's really nice seeing you though," she said.

"Are you sure? I mean, I'm starting to think that maybe you didn't want me to show up here like this."

"It's just a surprise, that's all."

"And obviously not a good one."

She looked at me carefully and took a swallow of her drink.

"It's a good one."

"So what's wrong then?" I asked.

"Nothing's wrong. Well, not really wrong. It's just that your being here is giving me all kinds of mixed emotions," she responded.

"What do you mean?"

In the silence that followed my question, I could have died a million times. I tried to fix my gaze on her and will her to speak, but her patience wore me down. What little control I had over the conversation evaporated in the time it took her to open her mouth and speak again. This was clearly her show, and I was along for the ride.

"A lot's changed since the last time we were together," she said slowly.

"Are you seeing someone new or something?" I asked, fully aware that this was the greatest of the probabilities.

She lowered her head, losing herself in the slight swaying of the Smirnoff bottle in her right hand. "No. I'm not involved with anyone anymore."

A strange feeling came over me as I digested the weight of her words. Clearly there was someone after me, but it seemed as though that experience had taken a toll on her. I wanted to ask about what had happened while I was away, but I knew that it was better to leave our pasts behind us if we were going to move forward.

I reached over across the space between us on the sofa and rested my hand on her leg. She placed her hand over mine, and I half-expected her to remove it, but she didn't.

I carefully crafted my next words and began: "Hearing your voice again after all of this time has been one of the most beautiful and unexpected things to happen to me in quite some time."

At this comment, she smiled and rubbed her hand across mine. My skin tingled from her touch, itching and aching to be rubbed by her delicate, yet strong fingers.

I continued, "I just wanted to know if we could be together again. Serena, I love you."

She lowered her head and turned away from me. Raising a hand, she brushed it across her eyes, leaving the traces of tears along her face and hand.

In her silence, I felt prompted to ask how she felt. "Do you love me?"

She turned to face me, and looking deeply into my eyes, she nodded her head. "Yes. I love you."

"Then what's wrong? Did I upset you?"

"No."

The word was so soft that I found myself leaning in to catch the syllable as it brushed across her lip. My lips touched hers, and we kissed each other briefly. As she stopped and leaned back, I edged forward, kissing her again. This time my tongue found its way through the space between her lips, and I felt her tongue meet mine.

No sooner than the kiss began, it ended with her pushing her hands into my chest, moving me back to my side of the sofa.

"What's wrong?" I asked again, starting to become irritated by her lack of forthrightness.

"A lot's changed since the last time."

"Like what?"

Her next words fell into the vacuum of silence in such a way that they were suspended in mid-air. "I'm HIV positive."

For a moment I didn't even register her comment in my brain. I just stared at her in utter shock. Slowly the nature of the situation dawned over me as I found myself mumbling those three letters. Then I felt my own stomach plummet as I realized that she had to have contracted it from somewhere. *Was it me? Was I HIV positive and didn't know it?*

Reading my mind, she spoke again, breaking the silence that followed her initial comment. "I got it a little over a year after you left. I had been dating this guy named Torrance. He found out that he had gotten it from an earlier relationship and didn't know it. He told me that I should get tested. Shortly after I found out that I was positive, he moved back to his hometown in Ohio. He wanted to be at home if he became sick."

She took another long sip from her Smirnoff Ice and continued. "I got so depressed I almost took a bottle of sleeping pills. I just wanted out. I really wanted out. But as I sat there writing my letter and getting ready to take my pills, I just realized that I wasn't ready to die. Not like that. There were still things I wanted to do in life.

"When you got back in contact with me, I had gotten used to living each day to the fullest. That's why I opened up to you so quickly. That's why I told you how I felt about you. I have never loved anyone the way that I love you, and I know that I will always love you, regardless of what happens to us."

"Man," I sighed. I didn't know what to think. My mind was in a deep haze, and as I sat on the sofa, it felt as though my body was completely numb.

"I was going to tell you soon. We were just starting to get reacquainted, and we hadn't gotten to the point where I felt comfortable telling you that. I had no idea that you would pop up here on my doorstep. I would've never wanted you to find out this way."

I opened my mouth to speak, and I was surprised when my voice choked in my throat and my eyes became glassy. I realized that I didn't really know what to say, so I reached out my arms to her and took her warmly into my embrace. I held on to her as if letting go would cause my body to collapse.

"It's okay," she whispered repeatedly in my ear. "I'm going to be okay."

When I finally released her, my face felt like it had been lifted to the sky during an April shower. Tears collected along my jaw line, and she brushed them away with her hand. In my feeling of hopelessness, I failed to recognize the immediate irony of her gesture: I was the one who was crying this time, not her.

"I love you," I told her.

"I know," she responded.

We sat in silence for a moment. I had not decided how long I would stay in New York when I arrived, and I didn't know what to do at this point. We could go on being friends until we could be friends no more, and I could return to the safe confines of my own Californian existence, or I could stay in New York indefinitely as I planned my next move.

"You're welcome to stay the night," she said.

"Whoa! Are you kicking me out tomorrow?"

I had already concluded that I would be staying the night with her, so when she couched the statement in those exact words, I knew that there was something more to it.

"I'm not kicking you out. You know I wouldn't do that. But I think you should get on back to California. I know that this is a lot to digest and that you probably need some time to yourself to take this all in."

She placed the empty Smirnoff bottle on the coffee table in front of the sofa.

Although she had a point, I wrestled with her on leaving so soon. She told me that she had an audition for a play the next day and that she would be singing at a wedding the day after. In other words, there was no need for me to stick around.

"What about us?" I asked. The question had been looming beyond the horizon the entire evening, and now it was out there, a living, breathing thing.

"Can't we just be happy in knowing that we love each other without needing to rebuild a relationship around it?"

"But I want you."

"Kyle, don't you see? I'm HIV positive. This can't work. It just can't!"

I dropped my head. "But I love you."

She stood up slowly from the sofa and looked me in my eyes.

"You're a sweet man," she said, as she walked back to her bedroom and closed the door.

Alone in the room, I reclined on the sofa and gazed up at the ceiling. The whole evening had been surreal. I could not believe that I had jumped on a plane so quickly to come to New York. I also could not believe that everything she told me was real, although I knew deep down that she had no reason to be dishonest with me.

I closed my eyes, locked in thought, and found myself reflecting. I relived the moment that I saw Serena, as she stood singing on the stage of that Brooklyn poetry club. I remembered that first conversation, that first date, that first kiss. I relived dancing with her against the skyline of the city as her band members played beautifully in the background. I relived leaving her, and I relived that pain and anguish of not having her in my life any more. But here she was telling me that she was sick, and that she was not willing to chance another relationship with me. A dull ache spread throughout my body.

I rose from the sofa and went to her bedroom door, knocking gently.

"Come in," she said so softly I could barely make out the words.

I walked into the dark bedroom, removed my shoes, and lay down on the queen-sized bed next to her. My arm moved around her waist, and she laid her arm over mine.

We didn't speak, but I held her tightly until we both fell asleep.

...

The next morning, Serena arose early and began to prepare to leave for her audition. I decided I would leave the apartment when she left for her errands.

Standing in front of the brownstone that housed her apartment, I was at a loss for words. She placed her arms around my waist and leaned into me, hugging me with all that her small frame could muster.

"I'm coming back," I said matter-of-factly.

She just looked at me.

"I want to be with you and be here for you."

"You don't have to do that," she said.

"I know, but I want to. You're the only one for me. And I don't know how all of this is going to work out, but I'm willing to try."

She looked up at me, and I held her face, kissing her gently on the lips.

"Okay," she said softly.

"Okay?"

"Okay."

She released me, and I walked with her to hail a cab.

"Good luck on your audition," I said.

"Thank you. And you have a good flight."

I leaned over and kissed her again.

"I'll call you tonight when I make it back, and I'll start looking for another flight to come back in a few weeks. I have to tie up a few things before I come back."

A smile spread across her beautiful face. "Okay."

A cab pulled up to the curb down the street from the brownstone, and I opened the back door for her. As she set one foot into the cab, she turned back to face me.

"Thank you for coming," she said.

"I'll be back soon. I promise."

"Okay."

The cab pulled off slowly, and I walked down the block to hail another cab to get to the airport.

...

Shortly after my plane touched down in San Jose, I called Serena to let her know that I had arrived. After several rings, the voicemail came on prompting me to leave a message.

"Hi, baby," I said. "I just wanted to let you know that I made it back to San Jose. I'm about to catch a cab to the house. Give me a call when you get this message. I love you."

I hung up the phone, a smile spreading across my face. Although I tried to conceal them, my lips spread apart and my teeth came blazing through as if I were being asked to pose for a photograph on "Picture Day" in grade school.

When I returned to my apartment, I unpacked my duffle bag and put on Chaka Khan's "Through the Fire." As the melodies and lyrics wafted, I found myself completely lost within the song. As cliché as it might have sounded, the song allowed me to imagine us running towards each other across beautiful green meadows punctuated by the yellows, reds, blues, and purples of a thousand flowers.

I reclined on my bed, losing myself in the music as I stared at the ceiling. I hoped to be out of my apartment by the end of the month, and I could not wait to be next to Serena again. I wanted to hold her and let her know that we would fight this thing together, that I was prepared to be all that she needed me to be.

As the night began to draw to an end, I picked up my cell phone to check for any messages I might have missed due to a momentary signal loss, which I knew was always a distinct possibility given the location of my apartment. The signal was strong, and there were no messages. I called Serena again. The phone went straight to voicemail, so I left another message.

Turning off the lights, I returned to my bed and lay down on my back, my cell phone resting on my chest set to vibrate when she called. I closed my eyes, and fatigue settled over me like a silk shroud. Within minutes, I drifted off to sleep.

I awoke around three in the morning and immediately checked my phone. The signal was still strong, and there were no messages. I didn't know why I had been so anxious to hear from her, but I felt as if seeing her had awakened something in me that had been dormant since I left New York. Patience was something that I no longer felt the urge to muster. My feelings were immediate, as was my need to express them.

After reluctantly returning to my slumber, I awoke around noon to a still apartment, sunlight trickling through my partially opened blinds. After checking my phone, I decided to walk over to the gym and work out for a while to free my mind from the prison of worry over Serena calling.

After an hour of pressing, pulling, and curling weights, my body stiffening with soreness. I returned to my apartment determined not to focus on my phone not ringing. The day passed along quietly, and by the following morning, I decided to call her apartment again. When the voicemail came on, I immediately hung up the phone and dialed up the New York City Police Department.

After being shuffled through the switchboard, I was finally connected to someone who was able to send a patrolman around to check Serena's apartment to make sure everything was all right. I left my number for someone to call in the event something turned up.

An hour later my phone rang. After having sat quiet for two days, the ring startled me. I ran into my bedroom to retrieve the phone from the bed, quickly scanning the caller ID. When I saw that the number was a New York number, I held my breath hoping to hear Serena's voice.

"Hello, may I speak to Kyle Taylor? This is Officer Madeline O'Keiffe with the New York Police Department."

"Oh, hi. This is Kyle."

"Mr. Taylor, I just wanted to let you know that we dispatched a unit already in the neighborhood to the address you requested. A Miss Serena Daniels answered the door and appeared to be in no distress. We notified her that we had been asked to look in on her and see if everything was all right. She told us that she was fine."

"Oh. Thank you. I appreciate your checking it out."

"No problem, Mr. Taylor."

As I hung up the phone, I sat down wearily on the edge of my full-size bed. I couldn't understand why Serena hadn't called me. Maybe I was just being paranoid; after all, she had informed me of her busy schedule before she left for the audition. At least I knew that she might still be in her apartment since the police had just left. Also, she had to have known that I was the one who sent the police to her apartment. I picked up my cell phone and dialed her number again.

The phone rang and rang until the voicemail picked up. Flustered, I left yet another message and hung up.

For the next few days, I resigned myself to the fact that I would never hear from her again. Her words seemed so empty as I replayed our last moments together. I felt forced to confront the issue of whether or not I had misread the signals.

It seemed clear that in the time between the moment she stepped in that cab and the moment I arrived in San Jose, something had changed. And whatever it was that had changed was haunting me with a silent vengefulness.

...

In the end, I never returned to New York.

I accepted a job offer with a small technology firm in the San Jose area after I finished my degree. It took me a while to get over Serena, and I felt as if I crashed much harder this time around. I don't know if it's because of love and the sensation of having found the person whom you believe is "the one." It could very well have been that I felt I had an obligation to somehow rescue her from something that no one could or maybe rescue her from the pain I imagined that she was experiencing. Then it occurred to me that it could have been me who had needed rescuing, not her.

Maybe it was one or all of those things. But maybe, just maybe, it was that eerie sensation of there being no closure that propelled me to fall so low this time. It seemed next to impossible that I could move forward in my social life without having an understanding of what went wrong.

The closest I came to a resolution was three months after what I would later recognize as my final visit to Serena's apartment. Tucked in with miscellaneous bills and my monthly issue of *Uptown* magazine was a postcard of The Apollo Theater in Harlem. The postmark was from a New York City zip code. There was no return address. Only a simple phrase written in familiar penmanship danced across the page, lapsing into ellipses: *I couldn't....*

I tacked the postcard on the wall of my bedroom, and on the rare occasion these days when I become saddened by the hand life has dealt us, I attempt to fill in the ellipses of the card with my own dreams of us dancing together again — should we share another lifetime.

When HIV Is a Livable Condition with Condoms: Work It Girl

Randall Horton

new-love wearing logical rouge lipstick conceptually sashays,
illogical would be too ignorant a testimonial when strolling
stiletto heel pumps against the grain of traffic—an illusion, is art
magicians never predict, what's under the skirt, make-believe
tina turner legs present an optical illusion—:
under a chandelier of bright moon, winos howl perfectly
at night, the peter can't see straight phallic tendencies or won't
nobody challenge hocus pocus power, the new in love
traditionally, men & women do not blur boundaries
to overrule wall paper painted blue
little boy loving pink learned pugilism, to survive
who you calling sissy ass muthafucka new-love dot eyes, amazed
at the I in he she or them, few understand the muscle of I *am*
like code switching down logan circle could have been a runway.

Your Style

Solmaz Sharif

lime tie popping off the ice white button down
stiff collar dark wash denim your feet high-fiving the pavement
your burnt sienna blazer vintage store find
your bedroom walls painted blue with green
and yellow stripes but standing in the Target
bedstuff aisle i can't figure out what kind of pillowcases to buy you
now that you need four more pillows to compliment the four
already on your queen bed to cushion your bones
there is no meat left on your body
all shitted away you joked ahmed said you had lost weight and
when a gay man says you lost weight then something's going on
i snorted called it stress i also need to pick you up a new
preferably heathered grey thermal small or
extra small now that you can't do the laundry now
no flesh insulates your bones against this bay area winter
also new boxers for aforementioned reasons
i will buy the boudoiritries and walk them over
to your tenderloin apt make your bed after you grunt and pull
yourself off it the low water pressure of a shower battering
your skull sends you into a pain so great you're telling me about it
i struggle over what color pillowcase is appropriate now
that i think you are dying i am itching to leave your house and
you have already begun to say things like
i know you have your own life and other things you have to do like you will say
from your bed one week later when i visit you in Kaiser
and a month after that when you call to warn next visit i make
i will have to wear a face mask

sanitize my hands before i enter your room
you don't tell me yet that there is one
t-cell left in your body or about the nurse slipping brochures
regarding god's wrath against fags in your hospital drawers
you never ask me to wear a mask
you initiate every hug as i leave your hospital door
even though my petri dish of a body could set off
a wildfire through your bare branched frame
you hold me as you always live your life knowing
love can kill you and still loving first
still loving hard

A Way to Get Born

Keli Stewart

"You are my child; that is why I let you suckle at my breast."

—Lady of Waters

grandma tied a towel around my belly, tight enough to girdle blackened stomach. *breasts too ,to get the milk out.* she smiled, folded me like a sheet or a soldiers death flag. cotton. creases. kin. this is how she would prepare my body. i'm a swaddled baby, a woman in a ghost sheet, sexless, breasts collapsing underneath gauze, milk pushing through. my soiled spots look like buttons of spray-paint. i want us touching. i want him to feel his mama. when i hold him, he roots at my wish breasts. i feel his mouth against curd.

Blood Mother

Terry Dugan

We dance in a circle,
Your pink parka
stuck halfway up your spindly arms.
Santa's outside, I say softly.
The squirming stops,
coat slides off with a final yank.

You look askance at Santa
when he bursts through the door.
Tall, skinny, sweating,
covered in cheap red flannel
wispy white nylon beard.
He does his best *ho, ho, ho*
Have you been a good girl?

I see in your raven eyes
this Santa is all wrong,
stethoscope dangling from his neck
Vacutainer tubes sticking out of his belt.

You forget puzzlement.
Squealing, you reach for
the green foil package he offers,
shiny portal to wonder and awe.

But you're right as usual;
humming "Santa is coming to town"
he has an agenda:

asking if you gained weight,
peering down your throat
with a flashlight and a stick.

I try to distract you
with promises of cookies and cake,
candy canes and coca cola.
But your antennae are twitching.

Like you didn't know
they were starting an IV
when I tried to carve
a Halloween pumpkin with a hypodermic.

Or when you stared listlessly at
papier-mache pilgrims pinned to
your crib while you ate
turkey and trimmings through a feeding tube.

Help me, Santa pleads.
What kind of Santa is this?
What kind of mother
exposes her baby's veins
averts her own gaze
listens impassively as you cry,
prays blood will come
fast and fulsome.

Chimayo

Christopher Woods

After we had driven through Talpa, the air seemed to turn cooler. The road climbed towards the near, somber grey clouds. In the mountains I saw blue mists clinging to ridges and layering in the high valleys like fallen smoke. On the road to Chimayo, we were also on the road into darkness. Not the sadly familiar dark of night, but in that special way that light itself can be pressed out of life.

How can I tell you all this without explaining our state of mind, how we were filled with equal amounts of hope and doubt, each battling the other for the upper ground?

All we could be certain about was the road itself, and where it would take us. How we came to be on that road, the one leading to Chimayo, was of course a different matter. The reasons were many, as were all the people and places along the way. And by this I do not mean rivers crossed, or the simple adobe houses nestled in the valleys of firs, or even the languid cows on steep slopes that seemed to reach all the way to heaven.

I can tell you about the road to Chimayo. I can tell you about other roads. But no matter what I say, there will be no changing the reason why we went to Chimayo. Not hope or prayer or doubt can change a thing. Chimayo waited for us as it had waited for the others. It waited for Lenny like it did all its supplicants. And Chimayo, my friend, is very patient.

I remember that we did not talk much. I wondered which was more deafening, the silence in the car or the landscape itself. Once, when it was raining, Martin and I saw a white horse standing in an open field.

"Make a wish," he told me.

"But why?" I asked.

"Always make a wish when you see a white horse," he said.

I knew something about wishes and when to make them. Seeing a loaded hay truck groaning down a road or to the pagan deities residing in rainbows. When tossing a coin into a fountain, or down a well. But I had never made a wish when seeing a white horse.

"You're going to Chimayo and you won't make a wish on a horse?" Martin asked.

"Go on, damn it! Make a wish."

I watched the rain. The field and the horse were both gone now, but I did it. I made my wish. And when I was finished, I felt no different. I looked in the backseat to check on Lenny. It was obvious he had missed the white horse.

Lenny had slept most of the way since leaving East Texas. He was on the downside, we knew.

Others, our friends, had gone the same way. But as Martin had already pointed out, twice, none of our other friends had been to Chimayo.

Early on, I had mixed feelings about going. I knew nothing about shrines except for pictures of Lourdes and Fatima I had seen in magazines. To me, they were as distant in concept as they were in miles. Certainly, no one I knew had ever gone to a shrine to be cured, of anything. I was sure that shrines were the most desperate places on earth. They would need to be just to exist at all, to lure the damned who were left with nothing but faded dreams and tattered scraps of faith. And I also had mixed feelings about faith.

Martin wasn't familiar with shrines either. But when I called and told him that Lenny wanted to go, he quickly agreed to drive us there. Lenny was our friend. There wasn't a lot we could do for him but try to honor his wishes. There was another side to this as well. Martin and I hoped that other friends would do the same for us if needed.

Earlier, Martin had said something about the banquet of years and how the table was being cleared earlier than anyone could have imagined. But it was not until we were sitting in a McDonald's, in Wichita Falls, that I truly understood what he meant. All the McPeople! By then I had begun to notice how all the people working behind the counters, as well as the customers themselves, all looked alike. And I realized they looked alike because, for them at least, the banquet of years was still in progress. Not so for our friend, Lenny. Once, when he was asleep and his talk betrayed delirium, I became worried.

"He's getting worse," I told Martin.

"I know," he said, his eyes staring straight ahead. "But we have to keep driving."

"But what if something happens," I ventured, "out here, on the road?"

"It can't," he said, a wild kind of faith in his voice. "Hasn't Lenny had enough thrown at him already? No, he deserves to get to Chimayo."

Lenny dreamed his way across the border into New Mexico. It was night. I watched the stars, which had now become very bright in the wide, ebony expanse of sky. And I watched the white spine of the road, thinking of all the roads that had brought us to this one.

It was early morning when we reached the town of Chimayo, but already the famous church was open. Small groups of people, families most likely, milled about outside beneath the trees. Nearby, a small creek trickled noiselessly across flat rocks. After combing Lenny's hair, Martin and I helped him into the church.

Inside, it was deathly quiet. The only discernible sound I heard was that of rosary beads clicking, moving through earnest fingers. Then, as we waited our turn to enter the shrine behind the altar, I could hear the sounds of footsteps coming and going. Some seemed certain, others more hesitant. Some were hurried, while others made slow progress, perhaps savoring the moment.

At last we were allowed to enter a small hallway that led to the shrine itself. The walls of the narrow passage were covered with canes and crutches, letters and photographs, statues, and relics. There were even some crudely made crowns-of-thorns, speckled with dried blood. Some had come well prepared, I thought. Standing in that hallway, we waited for our turn.

I looked at the faces of those coming out of the shrine room. Some people were wiping away tears. Others seemed to be making a supreme effort to retain their composure. I think that all of them, down deep, wanted to cry out in desperation against whatever unfairness had brought them to Chimayo.

But no one cried out. They knew that, by doing so, perhaps things would only worsen. In the end, all they could do was hope. Without that, without keeping on, they had nothing.

At last, we were allowed to enter the tiny room ablaze with the light of hundreds of candles. The heat was intense. I could see that the ceiling was low and black, but from the smoke or charred hopes I didn't know. On the floor was a hole with dirt inside it. The sides of that hole were scraped clean from anxious fingers.

We helped Lenny to his knees and watched as he felt at the edge of that hole. A weak smile on his face, he reached down into the hole with both hands. He grabbed fistfuls of dirt and rubbed it on his arms and face. Then, when he was done, we helped him to his feet again. He stood there silently, in that heat, his face was expressionless. I didn't try to talk to him. I knew he was thinking about time. If a cure were to come, how long would it last? And if it didn't come, what then?

All of a sudden, something happened that truly amazed me. Martin got down on his knees and did the same thing Lenny had done. I never expected it from him. When he finished, he remained there, kneeling. I had never seen Martin pray. When he finally stood up, I knew I had no choice.

I swallowed the scream that I felt rising in my throat. I knelt down beside that hole in the floor. I reach down into it as far as I could. I wanted dirt that no one else had touched. I don't know how long it went on, my frantic digging. At last Martin pulled me to my feet. I looked at my fingers, now caked with dirt. And, as Martin led me away, I saw the faces of the others, waiting for their turn.

In that church, I could see a desperate hate in their eyes. They were resentful because I had taken so long. As if another minute or two might make a difference for them. There was no way for them to know, of course. I didn't blame them. Suddenly, as we came into the bright sunlight outside the church, I felt ashamed of my greed.

Silently, I helped Lenny to the car. He walked so very slowly. Steps. One after the other. Wherever they would go, wherever they would lead us. Between my doubts and a faith in blessed dirt, I trusted my feet to find the path that would last the longest.

CJ 4321

Nina Bennett

The third time CJ
came in for an HIV test
it was positive. I paced
my office like a caged animal,
prepared to deliver his results.
He gasped when I said *CJ, your*
test is positive. Silent tears traversed
his downy cheeks as he shook his head.
How am I going to tell he whispered,
the next words nearly inaudible,
my mother?

He left, phone numbers for the HIV clinic,
support group, counseling hotline
stuffed in his jean jacket.
I filled out the standardized report.
Gender: male. Age: 22.
Mode of transmission: I searched
for a place to write luck ran out
but health department forms, unlike
election ballots, don't permit
write-in votes.

That night I eat dinner with my sons;
while they talk about school,
math tests, band practice,
I picture another son

who sits with his mother, stares out
the dining room window at purple finches
and cardinals, struggles to begin
an impossible conversation.

carrot juice

Clara Nura Sala

for Robbie

we squatted on a hostel roof
wrapped in worn blankets
under the sky's deepening meditation
under intersecting clotheslines
damp towels hung
above scattered sleeping bags scaled with frost
I wondered what dragons would emerge
fire and red with dawn

you slid the towels together around us
awkward terry cloth cave
moist whiffs of cheap soap and sunburn
you said it was intimate
I said it was claustrophobic
I pulled the towels apart with nervous fingers plopping like fish
in(to) night's vibrant spreading pond
fingers leaping to talk with you
the easy way, through stroke, caress (through caress)
I stuck out my tiny tongue to beg you for something edible, golden
your tongue brushed over mine   watercolors
oasis
my fingers
a wandering desert tribe   ate from the russet manna of your curls
your hands slipped under my ass
cupped both cheeks

cool white crocus bulbs transplanted
into two warm clumps of sod

I dipped one finger inside myself, ran it wet around the last flash of horizon
and Jerusalem was a wine glass full of ringing
I rolled another finger around your nipple
a concentrated child winding up a music box
you toppled naked beside me
I slid down lit with hidden gold
with wet reptilian wings

lost in your throat
I remembered what I had to say
as I tugged two towels open- "I'm HIV+," - closed -
"I'm totally healthy" -open - "it's only my T-cells"- closed
only my T-cells imploding
dead red/white dragons clogging my blood
universes extinguishing themselves
my lips faintly golden talked past you
to the ultraviolet backbone of dawn
held up my courage like a tent

quiet

no drunk stragglers stumbled/ing over bed rolls
no early rising hikers creaked/ing down stairs
a pair of lovers muffled thudding against the roof's far corner

you
said "drink more carrot juice"

stroked my hair
kissed me again,
and the morning star slid from the peace in my eyes
a kiss
four words:
juice
carrot
more
drink
poured around us like our four arms

and we fell asleep in
phrases paragraphs
planning our road trip for tomorrow
your dreamy hand tugging towels together to block out the new ache of light
my awakening hand parting them to see the horizon's singing pink aurora
raising the desert hills
red dragons flying

our mouths no longer press together
but
I drink more
my golden mouth
roaring out its chubby lion tongue
lapping up
sweet
orange
juicy
life

Absent Body

Richard Sawdon Smith

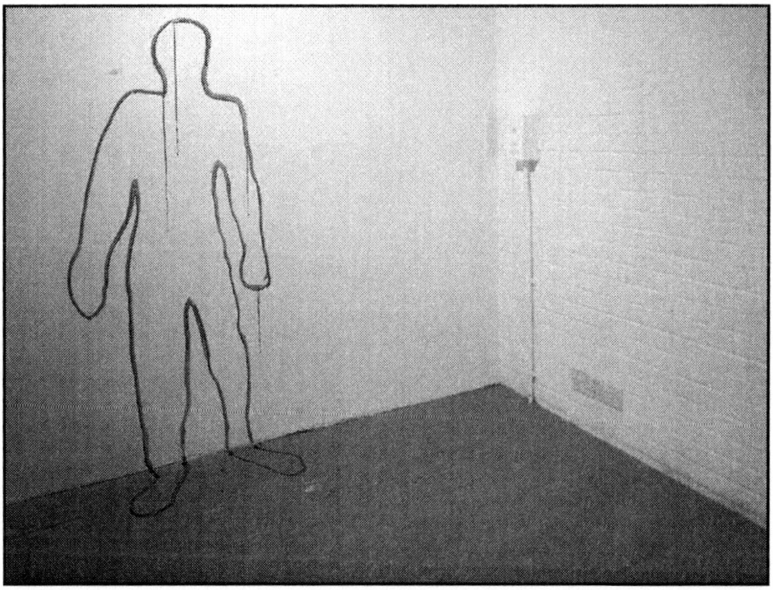

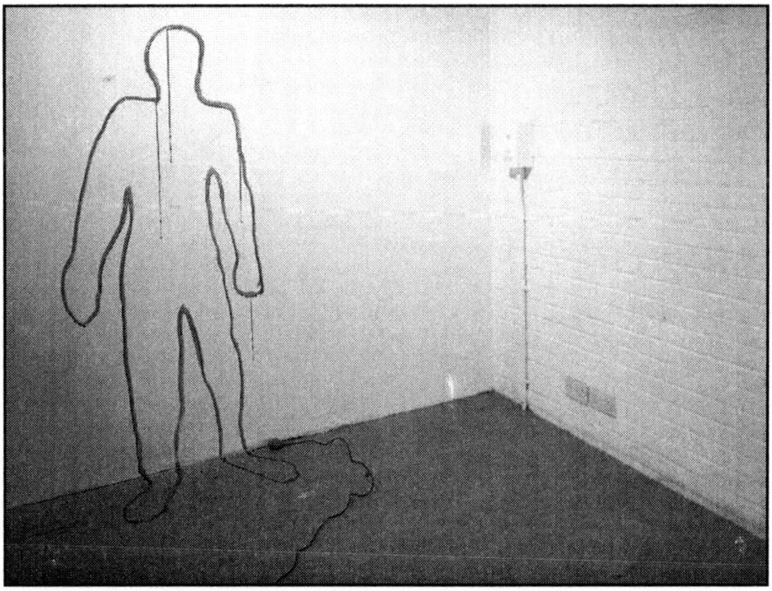

Contributors

Nina Bennett, author of *Forgotten Tears A Grandmother's Journey Through Grief*, is a Caucasian female who has worked in the HIV/AIDS field since the beginning of the epidemic. Born and raised in the Mid-Atlantic region of the United States, Nina was among the first in her state to be certified to perform anonymous HIV counseling and testing. She also served as a Buddy, facilitated a support group for people living with HIV, and worked as an HIV/AIDS case manager. Nina's poetry and essays have been published or are forthcoming in *The Smoking Poet, Philadelphia Stories, Pirene's Fountain, The Broadkill Review, Slow Trains Literary Journal*, the anthology *Mourning Sickness, Grief Digest*, and *Living Well Journal.*

Remica L. Bingham, a native of Phoenix, Arizona, earned an MFA from Bennington College and is a Cave Canem fellow. Among other journals, her work has been published in *New Letters, Callaloo, Gulf Coast* and *Essence.* Her first book, *Conversion*, won the Naomi Long Madgett Poetry Award, was published by Lotus Press and shortlisted for the Hurston/Wright Legacy Award. A book of her selected poems, *The Seams of Memory*, will be translated into Arabic and published in 2010 in conjunction with the Kalima Project. Currently, she serves as the Writing Competency Coordinator at Norfolk State University in Norfolk, Virginia.

Michael Boccardo is from High Point, NC, and publication credits include or are forthcoming in *The Bitter Oleander, Rattle, Poet Lore, The Asheville Poetry Review, Prairie Schooner, Eclipse, Southern Poetry Review*, and *RHINO.* He serves as an Editorial Assistant for *Cave Wall.* When not writing, he is a part time student and can be found lurking in the poetry section of the local Barnes & Noble bookstore where he is employed as a merchandise manager.

Michael Broder received his MFA from New York University in 2005 and is completing a doctorate in Classics at The Graduate Center of the City University of New York. His poems have appeared in *BLOOM, Columbia Poetry Review, Court Green*, and *Painted Bride Quarterly*, among other journals, and in the anthology *This New Breed:*

Gents, Bad Boys, and Barbarians 2, edited by Rudy Kikel (Orchard House Press, 2004). His essay on Sappho appears in *My Diva: 65 Gay Men on the Women Who Inspire Them*, edited by Michael Montlack (U. of Wisconsin Press, 2009). His current project is a dissertation on queer kinship and camp aesthetics in Roman satire.

Kwame Dawes was born in Ghana and raised in Jamaica. Dawes is the author of fourteen books of poetry and many books of fiction, non-fiction, criticism and drama; and editor of several anthologies of poetry. His collection, *Hope's Hospice*, appeared in the spring of 2009. In 2009, Dawes won an Emmy Award for the website livehopelove.com. He is Distinguished Poet in Residence at the University of South Carolina where he directs the SC Poetry Initiative and that university's Arts Institute. Kwame Dawes is the programming director of the Calabash International Literary Festival that takes place each May in Jamaica.

Terry Dugan is a former research scientist at the HIV Center for Clinical and Behavioral Studies at Columbia University School of Physicians and Surgeons. She began her 18 year career as a researcher for maternal and heterosexual transmission at Bellevue Hospital in the 1980s. She has published academic articles about AIDS and lectured about human rights and AIDS in Africa at Oxford University. Her poetry and fiction about the women and children at the Bellevue Pediatric AIDS clinic have won numerous awards. Her essay, "Saving African Women and Children One Movie at a Time: Truth Masquerades as Fiction" is in *Fingernails Across the Chalkboard: Poetry and Prose on HIV/AIDS From the Black Diaspora*. (Third World Press, 2007). She is working on a chapbook and a clinical memoir about women and children and AIDS in the 1980s.

Shanna Germain: Her award-winning stories and poems have appeared in *Absinthe Literary Review, American Journal of Nursing, Best American Erotica, Best Gay Bondage Erotica, Best Gay Romance, Best Lesbian Erotica, Blood Fruit: Queer Horror, Mediphors, Pulse*, and many more. Shanna is a white, bisexual female who grew up in the US but is currently living in Scotland.

Keith R. Green is a nationally recognized spoken word artist, HIV/AIDS activist, social justice advocate, and community journalist, hailing from Chicago's south side. As a Ronald E. McNair scholar of Northeastern Illinois University, he received an Advance Opportunity Fellowship to complete his Master's studies in the Mental Health concentration within the School of Social Work at University of Wisconsin-Madison. He currently serves as project director for Project PrEPare, a Chicago based research study that is exploring the acceptability and feasibility of Pre-Exposure Prophylaxis (PrEP) for HIV among young men who have sex with men. He maintains a regular column in the nation's most widely read HIV treatment education journal, *Positively Aware*, and has been a frequent contributor to both TheBody.com and Black-AIDS.org.

E. J. Guarino is an Italian-American author and educator who frequently writes about the indigenous art of the Americas as well as about travel and archaeology. His publications include *The Other Mexico: A Guide to Ancient Wonders and Modern Pleasures in Mexico.* His articles about Mexico, art collecting and Native American art and culture have appeared in *Mexico* magazine, *Native Peoples* magazine and in the magazine produced for the 2007 Heard Indian Market. He also writes a monthly column on Native art and culture for the King Galleries of Scottsdale web site. E. J. Guarino has recently completed *The Tongue*, a novel about the conquest of Mexico. He is currently finishing a novel on Motecuzhoma and is researching another set during Mexico's early colonial period.

Ellen Hagan is a writer, performer, and educator. Her work has been nominated for a Pushcart Prize, and can be found in the pages of *Failbetter, La Petite Zine, Check the Rhyme, 42opus, Submerged,* and *PLUCK.* She is a regular contributor to *Underwired* Magazine and was named a winner of the Next Great Writers Competition at the Carnegie Center in Lexington, Kentucky. Ellen is an Affrilachian Poet, and has received grants from Kentucky Foundation for Women and the GSA Toyota Alumni Fund. She is an Assyrian, Irish, Italian woman with roots in Kentucky and New York City.

Derrick Harriell received an MFA in Creative Writing from Chicago State University and is currently completing a PhD in Creative Writing from the University of Wisconsin, Milwaukee, where he teaches creative writing. His poetry has appeared in various journals, including *The Cream City Review, Reverie,* and forthcoming *Lamplighter Review* and *Dark Symphony*. Derrick also works as nonfiction editor for *The Cream City Review*.

Reginald Harris was a finalist for a Lambda Literary Award and the ForeWord Book of the Year for *10 Tongues: Poems* (2001). Recipient of Individual Artist Awards for both poetry and fiction from the Maryland State Arts Council, his work has appeared in numerous journals, anthologies, and other publications. A contributor to *Carry The Word: A Bibliography of Black LGBTQ Books* (2007) and *LGBTQ America Today: An Encyclopedia* (2008), he is currently completing work on two manuscripts.

Marguerite L. Harrold was born in Chicago at Cook County Hospital. Harrold earned her B.A in English from the University of Illinois at Chicago (UIC) and her MFA in Poetry from Columbia College Chicago in 2006. She currently works in HIV/AIDS Prevention for the Chicago Department of Public Health.

Beatrice M. Hogg is an African American woman who currently lives in Sacramento, CA. She has a BA in Social Work from the University of Pittsburgh and a MFA in Creative Writing from Antioch University Los Angeles. Her essays and poems have been published in several anthologies, magazines, newspapers and websites. She is currently working on a memoir, an essay collection and a novel.

Geoffrey D. Holman is a spoken word poet and the author of two collections of poetry and illustration (*Songs of Brick* and *Steel Giants and Ghettoetry: A collection of poetry & illustration*). Holman is a director and producer of many original stage plays as well as a visual artist. Born in Brooklyn, NY and raised in Deer Park, Long Island, Holman is a fourth generation artist.

Randall Horton is the author of *The Definition of Place*, and *The Lingua Franca of Ninth Street*, both from Main Street Rag. He is the co-editor of *Fingernails Across the Chalkboard: Poetry and Prose on HIV/AIDs from the Black Diaspora* (Third World Press, 2007). Randall has a MFA in poetry from Chicago State University and a PhD in English/Creative Writing from SUNY Albany. He teaches at the University of New Haven.

Christopher Jarred, originally from Detroit, moved to Chicago in 1996. His story is not one of fancy art schools or a child prodigy who began painting before he could walk. His is a story of pain, chaos, redemption and the search for peace and joy after the death of two wonderful parents.

Roopali Kambo is an artist based in Tallahassee, Florida and of Indian origin.

Basanta Kar is the author of two collections of poems, *The Naïve Bird and The Silent Monsoon;* Basanta Kumar Kar is Operations Director of Care India. He has written almost sixty five poems that meditate upon the real-life voices and stories of extremely disadvantaged women residing in various Indian states. His poems have appeared in a number of international and national magazines and journals like *The Houston Literary Review, Peril, Bewildering Stories, Smoking poet, Kritya, Tsar Books*, BBC, NDTV, UN Solution Exchange, Human Touch, EndVAW/John Hopkins , Peace and conflict monitor, Munyori, MOBIUS etc. Mr. Kar's vision is well recognized and he has the reputation of working in various international and national development organizations.

John Kotula is an artist and writer living in Rhode Island. He often writes about the ways in which people are impacted by art. He and his wife, Deborah Drew, were Peace Corps volunteers in Sonaguera, Honduras from 2005 through 2007. He considers his Peace Corps service to be among the best things he has done in his life.

Viet Lê is a Vietnamese American artist, writer, and curator born in Sai Gon, Viet Nam. Lê's artwork has been featured at DoBaeBacSa Gallery, Seoul; Sàn _rt Independent Art Space, Ho Chi Minh City; The Banff Centre, Alberta; Laguna Art Museum, CA, Cape Museum of Art, MA; Shoshin Performance Space, NYU; Highways Performance Space, CA, among other venues. His work has been published in *Fuse; Amerasia Journal; Art in Asia; West Coast Line; Crab Orchard Review; Newsweek Asia;* and the anthologies *Blue Arc; Love, West Hollywood; So Luminous the Wildflowers;* among others. Lê has received fellowships from Fulbright-Hays, William Joiner Center, Center for Khmer Studies, Fine Arts Work Center, and PEN Center USA. Lê recently co-curated humor us at the Los Angeles Municipal Art Gallery; and transPOP which traveled to Seoul, Sài Gòn, Irvine, San Francisco. He has edited special issues of *BOL Journal and Reflections: A Journal of Writing, Service Learning, and Community Literacy.* Lê received his MFA from the University of California, Irvine, where he has also taught Studio Art and Visual Culture courses. As a doctoral candidate at the University of Southern California, he is currently based in Phnom Penh.

Ghariokwu Lemi is a Nigerian artist and designer who is most renowned for providing many of the original cover images for the recordings of Nigerian musician Fela Kuti. His work involves a variety of styles, often using vibrant colours and individuated typefaces of his own design. More than 2,000 albums covers have been designed by Lemi, including covers for Bob Marley, E. T. Mensah, Osita Osadebe, Gilles Peterson, Miriam Makeba, and Antibalas. Many of Ghariokwu's cover images echo and sometimes comment on the work and politics of the recordings that they accompany, serving a consciously integrated metatextual function. Ghariokwu's work has attracted much attention in the West and is the subject of various retrospective exhibitions. His painting Anoda Sistem, created in 2002, is in the permanent collection of the Museum of Modern Art.

Toni Asante Lightfoot is a native of Washington, DC. There she was trained as a Civil Engineer at Howard University. She minored in Education and then decided to follow her heart to become a writer/performer. Lightfoot started teaching creative writing at Duke Ellington School of arts in 1994. In 1996, she joined the WritersCorp of America and taught youth and the elderly six days a week. In 2000, Lightfoot opened The Haven Bed & Breakfast Arts Retreat in Trinidad & Tobago. As the artistic director of The Haven, she set up workshops between artists in Trinidad and those from Canada, the US, and throughout the Caribbean, Africa, and South America. Lightfoot came to Chicago in 2002 after a stint in Boston as the artistic director of Blackout Arts Collective of Boston. She has performed her work on the CD *Some Nights* and was the voice of Ayisha Knight the first deaf poet on Def Poetry Jam. Lightfoot's work can be found in numerous anthologies and online. She is the co-editor of the Tia Chucha Press anthology *Dream of a Word.*

Melissa Lippard is a HIV counselor working at a community social service agency. Lippard writes a regular feature column for a food and dining magazine, and dabbles with the occasional poem. She has an MBA in nonprofit management and a BA in psychology and women's studies.

Michelle Mashon originated from New Orleans (the city that time forgot) and went on to train in Philadelphia in Illustration and Printmaking. She now lives in Chicago and found love in producing art events, exploring installation and performance art and creating new works. As an artist, she strives to expose the delicate rhythms and subtleties in the grotesque and perverse, and to explore the minor narratives lost in the bigger picture.

Tony Medina was born in the South Bronx and raised in the Throgs Neck Housing Projects. He served in the United States Army and earned a BA in English at Baruch College, CUNY, on the G.I. Bill. Medina has worked at Barnes & Noble Sales Annex, New York City Transit Authority, and has taught English at Long Island University's Brooklyn campus and Borough of Manhattan Community College, CUNY. The author of several books for adults and children, Medina's poetry, fiction and essays appear in over forty anthologies. Medina, whose most recent books are *I and I, Bob Marley* and *My*

Old Man Was Always On the Lam, has earned an MA and PhD in English from Binghamton University, SUNY, and is Associate Professor of Creative Writing at Howard University.

Kevin McLellan has recent or forthcoming poems in journals including: *Arch, Barrow Street, Drunken Boat, Exquisite Corpse, Hunger Mountain, Interim, Southern Humanities Review* and others. His chapbook *Round Trip*, a collaborative series with numerous poets, is forthcoming from *Seven Kitchens* (Spring, 2010). Kevin is a mutt with a Scottish last name and is from New Hampshire. Currently, he lives in Cambridge, Massachusetts.

Chloe' Yelena Miller received an MFA in creative writing from Sarah Lawrence College in May, 2005. She has poems published in *Alimentum, The Cortland Review, Lumina* and Privatephotoreview.org.

Gwendolyn A. Mitchell is a poet and editor. Her poetry has appeared in a number of journals and anthologies including *American Review, Prairie Schooner, Warpland: A Journal of Black Literature and Ideas* and *Essence* Magazine. She has conducted workshops in writing and literary arts, and in 2000, served as the first poet-in-residence for the Tougaloo Art Colony. She received her Master of Fine Arts in English from Pennsylvania State University. Ms. Mitchell is the author of *Veins and Rivers* and *House of Women*. She is the co-editor of two anthologies, *Releasing the Spirit* and *Describe the Moment*, both collections of literary work from Gallery 37 in Chicago.

Shahari G. Moore is the author of *It's Good Sunday* and the editor of ESSENCE Bestseller, *Violets: Inspirational Poems by the Women of Delta Sigma Theta Sorority, Inc.* and *Warpland: A Journal of Black Literature and Ideas*. As a multi-genre writer, she writes screenplays, live action-comedy, drama, creative nonfiction, and poetry. Shahari is a recent graduate of Chicago State University, where she earned an MFA in Creative Writing in May of 2007. She is also an alumna of Eastern Illinois University, where she earned a Master's degree in Educational Psychology.

Shahari is a recipient of the Kanye West scholarship for emerging writers and an alumna of the Nickelodeon Writers Lab at the American Black Film Festival, the Sea Island Writers Workshop on Sapelo Island in Georgia, and the Hurston-Wright Writers Workshop at American University in Washington, D.C. Shahari is a dedicated volunteer with the Writer's Guild Foundation of America West. She is tenured as an Assistant Professor with the City Colleges of Chicago in the Department of African American Studies, where she teaches Literature and Psychology. Shahari has studied abroad in Cuba, Morocco and Ghana. She is currently studying sketch writing at Second City in Chicago.

Alice Myerson is a nurse and a nurse practitioner and has worked in the trenches of the AIDS epidemic since the beginning. Her role has changed – it is to help young people learn to live with this virus rather than die from it. Although our ability to control the virus has improved, the devastation it causes to our young people and our community is profound as the disease continues to infect more and more young people every day.

Cyrille Phipps has been a media educator and video documentary maker for almost twenty years. She received a B.F.A. in Film Drama from Syracuse University and M.A. in Media Studies from The New School University. Recently, she was a Video Producer for Volume.com, where she was responsible for developing a comprehensive vision for video usage throughout the entire site. She has collaborated on various documentaries that have aired on PBS, TNT and the BBC. Much of her work has been featured in national and international festivals from New York to Hong Kong.

Victor Pond is an Afro-Latino and originally from the Republic of Panama where he obtained most of his formal education, including a degree in Psychology. Pond migrated to the US in 1981 and loved every minute of it. Currently he is a Consultant with ACRIA (AIDS Community Research Initiative of America) working specifically in a Health Literacy Program for Older Adults (over 50).

Ronnie Queenan is a fifteen year AIDS survivor. Realizing there is life living with AIDS. Painting is part of Queenan's healing and helps with getting in touch with being.

Mila Rozen has published articles for energy magazine – *Nafta&Gas Biznes* (Poland); as well as a short children's story in a an anthology by Muzyka and Duszy Gra. In 2006, when already a resident of England, Rozen worked as a researcher for established film directors and script writers such as Ken Loach and Paul Laverty and their highly acclaimed "It's a Free World" movie about immigrants living in Great Britain.

Rural Women's Health Project is passionate about educating communities about positive attitudes and behaviors. This project strongly believes that community members should play a role in building their own futures for a more sustainable health impact.

Chanell Ruth teaches English. She has served as Poetry Editor of *Warpland: A Journal of Black Literature and Ideas*; her poems have appeared in the *Louisiana English Journal*, *Fingernails Across the Chalkboard, Poetry and Prose on HIV/AIDS from the Black Diaspora* and the stage adaptation of the text in 2007. Her work was curated at the DuSable Museum in 2008.

Clara Nura Sala is a poet, educator and spoken word performer. Sala is a first generation American of Hungarian and German descent. Sala has been HIV positive since 1993. Sala's aim as a poet is to help others to heal by sharing her emotional and spiritual journey.

Solmaz Sharif was born in exile in Istanbul to Iranian parents. Sharif completed majors in Sociology and Women of Color Writers at U.C. Berkeley. While there, she studied and taught with June Jordan's Poetry for the People. She holds an MFA from New York University's Creative Writing program, where she taught creative writing and was a Goldwater Fellow. She currently lives in New York City.

Richard Sawdon Smith is a British photographer (b1963, England)) and an Associate Dean, Head of the Postgraduate School at the University for the Creative Arts, UK. He was winner of the John Kobal/National Portrait Gallery London Portrait Award 1997 and his photographs and writing are published in a variety of books including; *Cultures of Exile* (2004) Wendy Everett (ed); *Art & Photography* (2004) David Campany; *Pandemic: Facing AIDS* (2003) Umbrage Books; *Male Bodies: A Photographic History of the Nude* (2004) & *Fully Exposed: The Male Nude in Photography* (1990) both by Emmanuel Cooper; *Vile Bodies: Photography and the Crisis of Looking* (1998) Chris Townsend and *Representations of HIV and AIDS: Visibility Blue/s* (2000) Gabriele Griffin. His photography has been exhibited widely internationally.

Lamont Steptoe is an African American with Cherokee ancestry, born and raised in Pittsburgh, Pennsylvania. A graduate of Temple University, he is the author of twelve collections of poetry and the editor of two collections by South African poet, Dennis Brutus. Steptoe is the founder/publisher of Whirlwind Press, a Vietnam veteran, father and photographer. He is the recipient of an American Book Award, a Pew Fellowship in the Arts, two fellowships from the Pennsylvania Council on the Arts and an inductee of the International Hall of Fame for Writers of African Descent by the Gwendolyn Brooks Center at Chicago State University. His work appears in the *Longman/Penguin anthology of African American Literature* edited by Keith Gilyard and the Oxford University Press Anthology of African American Literature edited by Arnold Rampersad. His most recent books are *A Long Movie of Shadows, Crowns and Halos* and *Oracular Rumblings and Stiltwalking.*

Keli Stewart's work has appeared in *Meridian, Warpland: A Journal of Black Literature and Ideas, Letters To Fathers From Daughters, Torch Poetry* and *Calyx*. Her debut play "House of Forks and Knives," a play about identity, motherhood and a families battle with drug addiction, is the recipient of the Douglas Turner

Ward/Alice Childress Scriptwriting Prize. She is an MFA Creative Writing Student at Chicago State University.

Samantha Thornhill travels the globe performing poetry, delivering lectures, and facilitating writing workshops. Both a poet and published author, Samantha is a rising voice in the world of words. Her performance poem, *Little Odetta*, inspired by the late folk legend, is forthcoming from Scholastic Press in the form of a picture book. Also, her young adult novel *Seventeen Seasons* is soon to be published by Penguin Books. Samantha earned her Master of Fine Arts in poetry from the University of Virginia while coaching the VA slam team. In New York City she fulfills her position as poetry professor at the Juilliard School. She also serves as writer in residence at the Bronx Academy of Letters where she teaches creative writing and journalism courses to middle and high school youth. She is a native of Trinidad & Tobago.

Venus Thrash has had poetry published in *Gargoyle, Folio, Beltway Quarterly, Torch*, and the *Arkansas Review*, and in the anthologies *Gathering Ground*, and *Haunted Voices, Haunting Places: An Anthology of Writers of the Old* and *New South*. She has read at the Studio Museum in Harlem, The Schomburg Center for African American Research, and The Library of Congress. She earned a BA in Literature and an MFA in Creative Writing from American University. She is a Cave Canem graduate. She is an adjunct Professor of English at Trinity Washington University in Washington, DC. She meshes all sides of who she is into one body, mind, and soul in her poetry, and gives it form and meaning in her manuscript, *Womanology*, which speaks to audiences across all racial, gender, and sexual identities, symbolizing a living testament to and manifestation of those poetic ideals.

Ran Walker is an African-American male, born and reared in Mississippi (USA). A former practicing attorney, he is now a writer and English professor at Hampton University in Hampton, Virginia. He is the recipient of the 2005 Mississippi Arts Commission/NEA Fellowship for Nonfiction and a 2006 Hurston Wright Writers Week alumnus. His work has appeared in several fiction and poetry anthologies.

Nagueyalti Warren is a poet and educator from Atlanta, Georgia where she teaches African American Studies at Emory University and is a member of the Baobab Poetry Collective. Warren's second book of poetry, *Margaret Circa 1834-1858*, won the 2008 Naomi Long Madgett Poetry Award and was nominated for the Georgia Writer's Author of the Year Award. Also a Cave Canem fellow, her works have appeared in *Gathering Ground, the ringing ear: Black Poets Lean South, Essence* Magazine, *Pluck,* and *Drumvoices Revue.* Warren has edited the poetry anthology, *Temba Tupu! (Walking Naked) Africana Women's Poetic Self-Portrait* published by The Africa World Press, 2008.

Julene Tripp Weaver has lived in Seattle since 1989. She has a bachelor degree in creative writing from City University of New York, where she studied with Audre Lorde. Her Master degree, in Applied Behavioral Science, is from the Leadership Institute of Seattle. She worked in HIV/AIDS Services for 18 years. *Finishing Line Press* published her chapbook *Case Walking: An AIDS Case Manager Wails her Blues.* Garrison Keillor featured her poem, "Only What I Can Do," on *The Writer's Almanac.* Her poems are in many journals, three anthologies, and can be found online, some recent publications include: *Main Street Rag, The Healing Muse, Knock, Arabesques Review, Nerve Cowboy, Arnazella, Crab Creek Review, Pilgrimage* and *Letters to the World Poems from the Wom-Po LISTSERV.*

Keith Wilson is a Kentucky poet and recent Graduate of Northern Kentucky University. Many of his poems express his love for his family and explore his experiences as a biracial black/white man. His poetry has appeared in the journal *NKUExpressed* and *Appalachian Heritage.*

Christopher Woods lives in Houston and in Chappell Hill, Texas. He is the author of a novel, *The Dream Patch*, a prose collection, *Under A Riverbed Sky*, and a book of stage monologues for actors, *Heart Speak.*

jamila woods is a writer, poet, performer from the south side of Chicago. She has competed and performed in several slams including Young Chicago Author's Louder Than A Bomb inaugural college slam and the National Poetry Slam in 2009. She attends Brown University in Providence, Rhode Island and is studying Africana Studies and Performance Studies.

Emanuel Xavier is a poet, spoken word artist, author, editor, literary events curator, activist, and actor born and raised in the Bushwick area of Brooklyn. He transitioned himself from being a street hustler and a drug dealer to become one of the most significant and unlikely voices to emerge from the neo-Nuyorican spoken word movement using political, sexual, and religious themes throughout his work. He is of Puerto Rican and Ecuadorian ancestry. He has conducted spoken word poetry workshops and produced benefits and events for youth organizations throughout the country. His books include the novel, *Christ Like*, the anthologies, *Mariposas; A Modern Anthology of Queer Latino Poetry* and *Bullets & Butterflies; queer spoken word poetry*, and the collection, *Americano.*

avery r young, a performer and writer, has works published in *Fingernails Across the Chalkboard; To Be Left With The Body, Callaloo; AIMPrint* and other anthologies. His is also featured on several music projects.

Permissions

Remica L. Bingham, "The News in Spring" was published in *Conversion* (Lotus Press, 2007). Reprinted by permission of Remica L. Bingham.

Michael Boccardo, "The Closeness of Strangers" was previously published in the Fall/Winter 2006-2007 issue (#39) of *Hayden's Ferry Review.* Reprinted by permission of Michael Boccardo.

Gwendolyn Brooks, "The Second Sermon on the Warpland" and "Infirm" published in *Blacks* (Third World Press, 1987). Reprinted by permission of Brooks Permissions.

Kwame Dawes, "Quilt" and "Blouse and Skirt" both appear in the book *HOPE'S HOSPICE* (Peepal Tree Press, Leeds, UK, 2009). These two poems also appeared on the web site www.livehopelove.com—a site operated by the Pulitzer Center on Crisis Reporting. Reprinted by permission of Kwame Dawes.

Shanna Germain, Antibodies was originally published in *Pulse* magazine in 2008. Reprinted permission of Shanna Germain.

Viet Lê's artwork has been previously published.
Titles & previous publication info below:
untitled (faith), from the pictures of you series, 2002-2009
untitled, from the pictures of you series, 2002-2009
Chromogenic prints, Edition of 4 + 1 AP,
5 X 5 inches print (12 X 12 inches framed)
corpus, Vol. 3., No.1, Fall 2005. *Los Angeles and New York: The Institute for Gay Men's Health,* 2005. Reprinted by permission of Viet Lê

Ghariokwu Lemi, A.I.D.S.(Africa is Dying Swiftly) appeared in the catalogue of the exhibition titled *Black President: The Art and Legacy of Fela Anikulapo* (Palgrave Books, New York in 2003). Reprinted by permission of Ghariokwu Lemi.

Kevin McLellan, "Split Personality" earlier version published in *Barrow Street.* Reprinted by permission of Kevin McLellan.

Rural Women's Health Project, "Positive Voices of Dorm E" first appeared in *The Choice Is Yours,* (October 2007) a magazine developed in collaboration with Aid to Inmate Mothers (AIM), the Rural Women's Health Project, and the Alabama Department of Corrections Tutwiler Prison and the Alabama Department of Public Health. Funded by the Southern HIV/AIDS Prevention Initiative Pfizer, Inc. Reprinted by permission of Rural Women's Health Project.

Lamont Steptoe, "A Secret Code" was originally published in *Oracular Rumblings and Stiltwalking* (Whirlwind Press, 2007). Reprinted by permission of Lamont Steptoe.

Christopher Woods, "Chimayo" has in the *Santa Fe journal, Cezanne's Carrot,* Volume 1, Issue 2, (2006). A stage monologue version of "Chimayo" is included in *Heart Speak* and was produced in an all male monologue show of mine called *Lover, Killer, Amgel, Thief.* Reprinted by permission of Christopher Wood.

Emanuel Xavier, "Legendary" is from *Bullets & Butterflies: queer spoken word poetry* and the poem "Cielo" is from *Mariposas: A Modern Anthology of Queer Latino Poetry.* Reprinted by permission of Emanuel Xavier.

Acknowledgements

To the authors in this collection and to all who submitted pieces we are most humbled. You shared tremendous insight to the human experience around the sensitivity of HIV and AIDS. Special thanks go to Quraysh Ali Lansana, Tacuma Roeback, Tressa Jones, and Loren Buford for seeing this collection to light.

Special thanks to Toni Asante Lightfoot, Zahra Baker, C.C. Carter, the Center on Halsted (Chicago), and all of the wonderful participants from the Spring 2009 H.Y.P.E. Troupe.

This collection was supported by the Gwendolyn Brooks Center for Black Literature and Creative Writing, the HIV/AIDS Youth Prevention Education (H.Y.P.E.) program of the Gwendolyn Brooks Center, Illinois Department of Public Health, and the W.K. Kellogg Foundation.For all who are impacted and living with HIV and AIDS, *Spaces Between Us* lets us know we are closer than we think.

Ellis' Thank You's

First, to the many million gone. Ashe.

Many thanks to Quraysh Ali Lansana, Tacuma Roeback, Tressa Jones, and Loren Buford for making this project possible.

To my partner in crime, M.L. Hunter, you have taught me so much during this process. Thank you for your hard work, patience, and talent. I am ready for the next project. Are you?

To my friend and partner Kevin Baskins thank you for your support and love and thank you Naomi Zora for your unconditional love and sweetness while Mommy worked into the night. My sister Crystal Ellis thank you for telephone laughs. Ellis and Everett this book is for you and Naomi.

To Haki R. Madhubuti and the staff of Third World Press, I am always in awe of you. You are my word family.

To all the writers who are here in these pages and those who did not make it, I say thank you for believing in the healing power of words. Your words are the medicine. And always, my mama, Dr. Cheryl Slaughter Ellis. You have always filled the spaces. Thank you.

Hunter's Thanks You's

Peace and Blessings to my family (you know who you are) and my bois Jeffry Thigpen, Charles Braxton, and Keith Green—y'all support got me through. Rodney Pryor thanks for your pride and patience. Haki Madhubuti, Tacuma Roeback, and Randall Horton thank you for your votes of confidence and advice. Quraysh (Q, Professor, Prof Q), years ago you said I'm a poet and I believed and now learning the business of books — I thank you for allowing me to grow. Kelly (Dr. Ellis) out of all the years we've been around each other this has been the first project we have worked on together and the experience has been DY-NO-MITE! (Bring on more!) And to all that submitted and those who have been part of my literary growth — THANK YOU.

Editor's Bio

Kelly Norman Ellis is an associate professor of English and creative writing at Chicago State University. She is also the associate director of the MFA in Creative Writing program at CSU. She is a poet whose work has appeared in *Sisterfire; Black Womanist Fiction and Poetry, Spirit and Flame, Role Call: A Generational Anthology of Social and Political Black Literature and Art, Boomer Girls, Essence* Magazine, *Obsidian, Calyx, Cornbread Nation, Torch, Fire and Ink: An Anthology of Social Action Writing.* She is a recipient of a Kentucky Foundation for Women writer's grant and is a Cave Canem fellow and founding member of Affrilachian Poets. Her first collection of poetry *Tougaloo Blues* was published by Third World Press in 2003.

M.L. Hunter is a native of Indianapolis, IN via Lexington, MS (he thought he was born in Durant and Uncle Sam enlightened him when he joined the Air Force in 1989). Currently he lives in Chicago and received his MFA from Chicago State University in Creative Writing with an emphasis on poetry. He serves as the Communication and Policy Administrator for the Chicago Department of Public Health's STI/HIV/AIDS Division. Hunter has written for newspapers and magazines. He has served as Criticism Editor for *WarpLand;* co-editor for *Fingernails Across the Chalkboard: Poetry and Prose on HIV/AIDS From The Black Diaspora;* and co-writer for *Kevin's Room 3: Together.* Hunter is one of the co-founders of the HIV Youth Prevention Education (H.Y.P.E.), a project of the Gwendolyn Brooks Center for Black Literature and Creative Writing at Chicago State University. Hunter continues to work on his unfinished business in the manuscript, *Telling Secrets Backwards.*

Social Conscious III

Ronnie Queenan

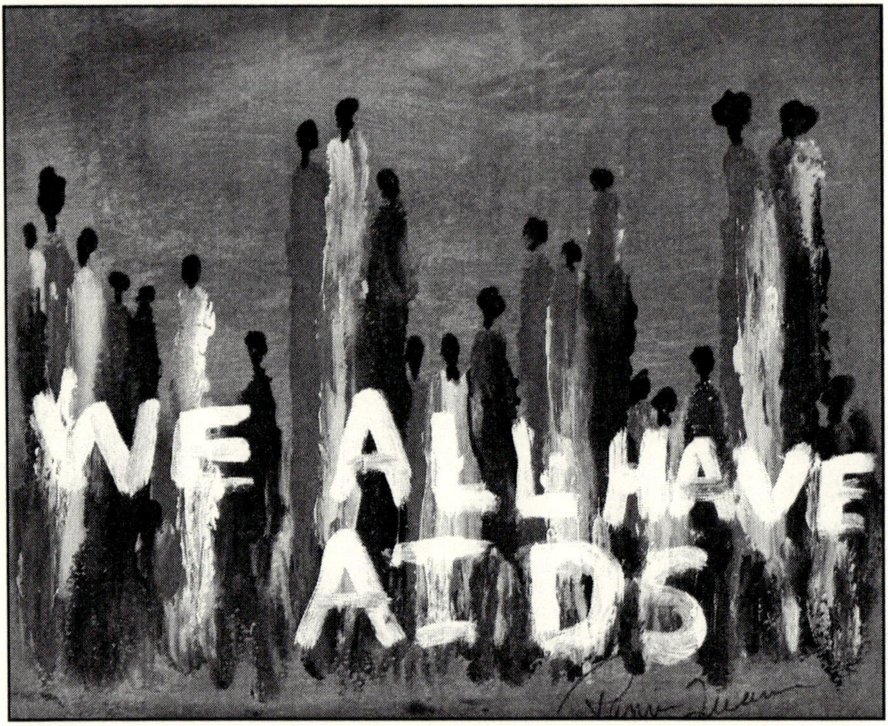

Infirm

Gwendolyn Brooks

Everybody here
is infirm.
Everybody here is infirm.
Oh. Mend me. Mend me. Lord.

Today I
say to them
say to them
say to them, Lord:
look! I am beautiful, beautiful with
my wing that is wounded
my eye that is bonded
or my ear not funded
or my walk all a-wobble.
I'm enough to be beautiful.

You are
beautiful too.